The Mystery of Health and Disease

The Mystery of Health and Disease

Why We Get Sick,
How We Can Reduce Illnesses
Lastly, Be Aware; It May Save Your Life

Hong Son Cheung

To order additional copies of this book, contact:
Xlibris LLC
1-888-795-4274
www.Xlibris.com
Orders@Xlibris.com
552704

Contents

To my respected and dearest mother

Madam Lee Tsing Chin

To remember her for imparting her cultural education to us

Also to my dearest father

Sir Cheung Mo Liong

To my dearest and respected brother

Mr. Christopher Cheung Hing Hung

To thank him for supporting our family in the earlier time
in our life

Also to my two dearest sons

Noland and Alvin Cheung

Preface

It is difficult for us, as human beings, to avoid health issues and diseases that occur in the body in one's lifetime. Even if this is true, however, no one really clearly understands the mechanisms of health and disease well now.

We all know what health is and what we could do to maintain our health.

For diseases, there are many different kinds happening to us, but no one really knows all the diseases clearly in the world. I don't know all the diseases; however, I know some of them.

I am not a doctor but had worked with a pharmaceutical company for thirty years until I retired in 1996. Therefore, knowledge was obtained from there during those periods. Also some different wisdom from thinking was collected later after I retired. It may be helpful for people to understand them for their health and might and could also solve their problems about sickness in their lives.

In this book, for easy to understand and also for general reader can read and understand its meaning. Thus, there are no medical and scientific terminologies in this book. Then, surely, it can help the reader to read, know, and understand this book not difficult. This book was written not for medical specialists. It's written in the simplest language to enable the general reader to read it. This was my goal for writing this book.

January 5, 2014

Willingboro, NJ 08046
USA

Acknowledgments

The author would like to thank those who supported him in writing this book. In alphabetical order, they were Alvin Cheung, Christopher Cheung, and Noland Cheung.

The author also would like to thank those who revised this book or pointed out potential issues with all kind suggestions. They were Alvin Cheung and Noland Cheung.

Chapter 1

Health

Health and diseases are important issues to humans. However, even most of us are aware and clear on the term *health*, but understanding the meaning of health is still a big question.

We all talk about health.

In medical society, Chinese and Western doctors, even including us, all know what is going on and understand about health. Thus, we always talk about health frequently.

Building up health means that after having the healthy body, we should get a good body. It sounds right to us, but in my opinion, it is not correct at all.

The reason is that we have found many humans with already strong bodies and good health. But it doesn't necessarily mean that those persons do not have diseases in their bodies. Vice versa, finding humans without diseases in their bodies does not necessarily mean they have a strong body and good health.

For this reason, even if we get strong, healthy bodies, we still have disease around. Thus, how can we conclude that we have good bodies?

If we want to achieve this goal, a good body, we should not only get a healthy body. It is certainly not correct and also not enough. We must also require "no disease (illness)." Certainly, we can reach and achieve this goal. After that, the body's good situation certainly could happen.

Now we understand, human just with health only certainly couldn't reach the goal to the good and well to our body. Certainly, it is not correct at all. It must require both situations, health and the absence of disease, happening together in human body there. Thus, after that, the body "well and good" could be achieved and could happen to us humans.

How can we approach the goal of having a true good, healthy body?

This is what we must do: make sure (1) that we have a healthy body and (2) that no disease happens in our body, together.

1. Make sure that we have a healthy body

    To have a healthy body requires you to do exercise frequently—at best, daily. Any kind of exercise would be fine, such as swimming, dancing, running, riding on the bicycle, climbing up a mountain, or working on the exercise machine. And even just walking would certainly be better than doing nothing at all.

    However, for doing exercise, there is one very important issue. It is more important than doing exercise. It is patience.

    Without patience, even if you do exercise for a while, you will quit it later on. You may do it again and quit again. By following this cycle, finally, the exercise would be stopped completely. This kind of exercise is no help at all. At the end, results happening from this kind of exercise surely must end up with nothing.

Therefore, in doing exercise, you certainly must also have patience together such that you can continuously do it frequently.

Doing exercise can surely make our body strong and healthy. But doing exercise could not by itself cure and take care of diseases.

Doing exercise can make our fighting ability stronger, promoting the ability of our immune defense system and also resulting in increasing the force level in our body. It also can make the environment around us change.

Thus, after the force (energy) level, fighting ability, and immune defense system are increased, our body should also feel much better and minimize or better prevent anything going wrong in the body.

This could be the reason why it makes us feel that doing exercise could help prevent and, thus as a result, cure and take care of diseases.

Let's take the hypothesis that the disease is still in your body.

Doing exercise is only making you feel better. If you're feeling better, then sickness should not be easily felt there.

2. Make sure that no disease happens in our body

   How can we prevent diseases from occurring in our body?

   If we expect not to get disease, first we have to know and understand why humans are sick and get disease.

   Why?

   I believe most of you asked these questions before:. Why do we get sick and have diseases? Is it life? Can those diseases that happen to us be cured and recovered from later? Are medical care and drug treatments necessary in life? I believe no one has the answer but will get it here.

   Why do we get sick and have disease?

   Sickness and diseases are certainly related and can occur in our body. However, our body is also directly involved and related to the environment presence. Thus, the environment should also relate to the sickness or disease that happened.

   Therefore, the environment may be considered as a reason to cause human disease or sickness. We used to live in this kind of environment. Our tendency would be to feel normal and happy and fit in (merge) with this environment. Therefore, certainly, this environment will be our living and natural environment.

   Our body, thus, will feel nothing wrong (no discomfort). Therefore, there is no disease symptom occurring. In case the environment changes, our body can't live and fit in or cannot adjust in this changed environment.

Uncomfortable conditions will occur in the human body under this changed environment; certainly, this will be responded to immediately by our body. Surely, we may have a different and potentially terrible feeling there. We can become sick. Sickness can occur from the change in the environment and what occurs in our body, which may cause an uncomfortable feeling. The uncomfortable feeling can be the occurrence of sickness. Thus the uncomfortable feeling is the sickness.

Environment

There are two different kinds of environments around our body. One is internal, and the other is external.

1. External environment refers to the natural environment from outside of our body. It is an environment (atmosphere) in the universe. It may also mean a big natural environment.

2. Internal environment refers to the environment inside our body. It refers to everything contained inside our body. It also means a small natural environment.

Both environments can cause us to become sick.

1. First, natural, external big environment

   This can include weather, temperature, cutting, hurting, viruses, bacteria, and so on—all are part of the natural (external) environment. All of them can result in diseases happening to us.

   As an example, the temperature dropped too low and is now too cold. It will result in you potentially having a headache, sickness, and maybe, leading to a disease. This is because of a natural environmental change resulting in you becoming sick.

However, this kind of disease is from the natural (exterior) environment *changing*; it certainly can be cured and one will likely recover. But recovery could happen under this condition: the environments *changing back* to the normal. Then this disease can certainly be recovered from. After the environment *changes back* to normal, uncomfortable feelings will disappear.

Thus, this sickness can lead to recovery. This uncomfortable feeling completely returns back to normal; the sickness is not present anymore. Then, it is not necessary to take drugs (medicine) and see the doctor anymore. This disease will be no longer there. Unless the environment goes back to the previous worse condition, the disease will not happen again.

Thus, this kind of disease results from the change to the natural environment (external). It can surely be cured and recovered at the environment's change back to normal unless the body is permanently badly damaged already by this. Otherwise, diseases will be fully recovered and gone.

2. Second, internal (small) natural environment

This is a very serious situation. Because this kind of environment occurs in our body, many things and materials are present inside our body. All those things are inside our body no matter what. The contents of the human body are required materials; we can't miss any one of them.

However, those things inside our body, we can't touch them easily or take them outside our body. But everything inside must be doing a specific physiological function for our body to maintain human behavior and life. Nevertheless *each thing must be present and must also be in a suitable amount (dose) in the body*. This is an important, valid rule for our body. We must keep this rule in our minds and understand that.

In some cases, the amount of anything changes from suitable to excessive in our body. Those higher amounts will result in a corresponding feeling as the environment also changes. Thus, its responsive physiological function is also changed to the abnormal behavior of our body. These changed situations will result in different feelings in our body too. This different feeling can be called or defined as sickness or disease to us. This will be explained later in the book.

Here is another question: how can it be that the amount of material inside our body changes from a suitable amount to more?

To understand this question, as an example, we eat meals every day to maintain our daily life. Suppose we eat two bowls of rice. After eating, later we must go to the restroom to excrete some waste food (feces) out of our bodies. Theoretically, we ate two bowls of rice, so the optimum amount that can be excreted out that must be also identical to the amount as we ate; it is two bowls of rice. Such as we only have $2,000 in our pocket. Therefore, the most amount of money that can be spent to purchase things from a store is also $2,000.

We understand this fact. However, in the situation, the amount excreted out from our body is not necessarily two bowls. It might be less than the optimal amount of two bowls from eating. Suppose the amount is only one bowl of rice excreted out, and thus, one more bowl of rice is found left over inside our body. This amount of one more bowl left in our body certainly contributes to the case that we talked above, how the amount changed to more in our body. If this condition happens every day, certainly, we should have many more bowls of rice remaining inside our body. This situation certainly is happening in our body by eating.

What will happen to us if there is an imbalance in our body?

Now if you take a total of forty bowls of rice at once, your body will notify you immediately. Your stomach feels so bad, and a terrible, uncomfortable feeling occurs there. This uncomfortable situation is surely from eating a total of forty bowls. It certainly contributed to the amount's increase occurring in the internal environment. Thus, we are sure that an imbalance inside our body definitely will result to an uncomfortable behavior (sickness or disease) happening in our body.

This kind of sickness comes from an uncomfortable (different) feeling, but this result's origin is from the environmental change, the amount increase or imbalance happened.

This explains why uncomfortable feelings happening to us can be called as sickness or disease.

We can use another example: if we drink forty cups of water at once. Water is different from rice. But forty cups of water inside our body also end up with a different uncomfortable symptom (compared with rice) happening in our stomach.

Both of those cases are from different foods; however, both end up indicating an imbalance with uncomfortable behavior or symptom. These uncomfortable situations and symptoms are completely different from each other. Even if different symptoms are indicated, they still are from the fact that an *excess* (of either rice or water) happened.

Water and rice are not the same and are different things.

Thus, water and rice would contribute different feelings; therefore, they would produce typical behaviors occurring in humans. Thus, the increased amounts from each of them should contribute different uncomfortable and nonidentical behavior (sickness or disease) in the human body. There would be a different sickness for each.

Thus, each individual, each thing, and each material in the human body—all of them—must follow this general rule. Each of them will have its own responsive function indicating its own behavior symptoms.

Thus, we can also conclude that if an amount of something increases in our body, it will result in having an uncomfortable symptom (sickness or disease) occur in our body. But what kind of uncomfortable behavior—what kind of sickness or disease, such as diabetes, hypertension, or others—can occur in our body? It is strictly depending on each individual.

Thus, the increased amounts only indicate that the uncomfortable symptom and sickness would occur. Which kind of uncomfortable behavior (which sickness or disease) happens is strictly decided by the kind of substance (material or food) in the body.

Is this symptom also truly occurring in the human disease?

We know these about some diseases:

1. If the sugar level is high in our body, it may result in diabetes.
2. If the salt level is too high in our body, it may result in hypertension.
3. If the cholesterol level is too high, it may result in a stroke or a heart attack.

The diseases (uncomfortable symptoms) above can result from the increased amounts of substances occurring in one's body. But which type of disease occurs is dependent on which type of substance (sugar, salt, and cholesterol, respectively) causes the condition.

In other words, we can hypothesize the following:

1. Symptoms of uncomfortable behaviors or feelings (sickness or disease) may come from an increased amount of a substance in one's body.
2. Which type of uncomfortable feeling (which sickness or disease) occurs is decided by the individual substance (in excess amount) in the human body.

Thus, it is possible that the increased amount of each individual material in our body will result in an occurrence of the disease (sickness).

When the amount of each individual substance increases, a corresponding disease would happen. There are many different individual substances in our body. If the amounts of each of them increases, certainly, each corresponding disease also occurs. Thus many different diseases will occur to us. This is the reason why humans have many diseases occurring in their body.

The amount, dose, and content (material)

However, the occurrence of disease is not only from the increased amount inside our body. It also can occur from decreased amounts inside our body.

For example, if you don't have enough sugar in your body, you will feel dizzy and uncomfortable. In this case, you just need to take a little piece of sugar to put into your mouth. The dizziness will probably disappear from your body. Thus, this uncomfortable feeling is resulting from a decreased amount of sugar in your body. Therefore, the decreased amount of substance will also result in having an uncomfortable feeling in our body.

Disease can also result from missing required materials or introducing a new material into the human body, but they will result in having a new different disease in a body.

For example, if we missed air in our body, we will die immediately. Air is a necessary material in our body. We can't live without its presence. Thus, it tells us that any required material missing from the body can result in a problem.

Introducing a new material component to the body, such as bacteria or viruses, the disease will happen to us. Thus, new material introduced into our body will also lead us to getting a new disease. Sometimes, they bring about serious effects to our life. We must be aware that new material should never be introduced into our body, especially new mutations of bacteria or viruses.

Some of these diseases have no cure and are deadly to our body because there are no drugs or medicines around to take care against these diseases. As far as we know and can find out, the fact is that many humans have died from this.

When a new drug can be found and invented in the near future, then these deadly diseases from mutant bacteria and viruses can thus be killed and cured. Until those times arrive, humans should still be very careful about them.

At the end of this section, we understand how diseases can happen to humans and also know that many diseases that can occur are from an incorrect eating habit.

Therefore, if we want to lessen the probability of having diseases occur, we must control our eating habits to eliminate those bad conditions.

1. Maintain the amount of everything at a normal level in the body.
2. Ensure that there are no missing things in the body and also that no new things are introduced into the body unless necessary.

Otherwise, disease would continue in our life. It is for our life, and it can't be cured and recovered from. It is because we can't easily touch inside our body to change those conditions back to normal. Thus, a doctor's care is required, and taking medication is also necessary in your life.

However, habits (including eating) are very hard to change for humans. Without changing, certainly, this goal is useless. The disease will be there as usual. Please do understand to change your life habits to help yourself get well. If you don't do it yourself, no one can help you except yourself!

Remember, when there are increased amounts of substance inside the human body, there is no easy way for us to take this excess out from our body. Diseases may occur. Changing habits and controlling ourselves are the only ways to fix this problem.

The concept for not getting diseases is already discussed above. The method to reduce (bring down to a lower amount level) those excess substances from the human body to the normal level is not talked about here. From the concept mentioned, I believe you will know how to control the level amount back to the normal.

Finally, to get a good and healthy body requires (1) building up a strong body and (2) not getting diseases.

They must be together, and it is not enough to have health alone.

Chapter 2

Diseases and the Heart

From now on, we will try to talk about diseases (sickness). There are so many diseases around. Practically, no one in the world understands all the diseases well. Therefore, there is no way to describe all diseases, one by one. Thus, the reason for diseases occurring is still not clear at all.

But as mentioned in chapter 1, the reasons for an imbalance leading to the occurrence of diseases are still true. Those reasons are (1) the amount of each thing is not at the normal level in the body, and (2) some materials are missing or new materials are being introduced into the human body. Those issues are still valid.

We don't understand how all diseases happen. Surely, we can't describe them one by one at this moment.

But the most common diseases—such as hypertension, diabetes, heart attack, stroke, three high, pain, irregular heartbeat, and so on—can still be described at the present. Those diseases are relevant to us and can be discussed here.

However, I believe almost all diseases are directly or indirectly from the result of eating. It can be from an increased or decreased amount in the human body and may also be from missing a required thing or the introduction of a new material into the human body.

Because all diseases may be a direct or indirect result from eating, it is, therefore, very important for humans to know heart issues here.

Before we talk about the heart

The question is, Why is it required for us to understand the heart, and how can the food get inside our body? Without knowing this, we have no way to understand how additional amounts affect us. Theoretically, food itself can't be absorbed and introduced inside the human body. Then, how can it enter the human body? The reasons are these:

1. We know that all food is big—big molecules, big particles, and big pieces. They all are big in size. Therefore, because it is big, it can't enter the human body and be absorbed.

2. There is also no hole at all in our digestive system, such as the intestinal organ, to allow the food to enter the human body.

After being eaten, the food that enters our body must overcome the above conditions.

After eating, because food is big, the mouth and teeth must chew this food first. Then the size of the food is thus broken down to a smaller size in the mouth. Besides that, there are some machines (enzymes) found in the saliva in the mouth. Those machines can further break down this smaller size to an even smaller size. Thus, those smaller-sized by-products from these steps then enter the stomach for further treatment. In the stomach, there is acid.

Acid. We know there are many kinds of acid, such as sulfuric acid, hydrochloric acid, and nitric acid. These all are strong acids. On the other hand, carbonic acid is a weak acid. There are also many other acids around.

A strong acid is powerful acid. They can break, denature, and destroy most materials easily, sometimes even metals. Our skin and muscle can be damaged in no time at all if touched by these strong acids.

The broken-down by-products of food from above then enter the stomach.

Hydrochloric acid is classified as a strong acid, and it is present in our stomach. Thus, this stomach acid (hydrochloric acid) is powerful enough to further break down those already smaller particles to even much smaller pieces.

After the step of stomach treatment, food then enters the intestine and also goes through some treatment there.

In the intestinal system, there are also other kinds of machines (enzymes) present that perform a further breakdown job there too. The force from intestinal movement can result in further reducing for those already small sizes to even much smaller. After all these steps are done, food becomes the very smallest size and can also enter the inside of the human body through the intestinal organ.

After treatment with all these steps, the food is changed to many different materials but can be classified in three different major groups.

1. Oil-like substance group (soluble into oil)
2. Water-like substance group (soluble into water)

3. Insoluble substance group (not soluble into either oil
    or water)

After treatment through all the steps from above, the question
then is how the food can get inside the human body, because
there is no hole there to allow this smaller-sized stuff to get
into the body.

To understand it

In our intestinal organ, we have three major parts that
function to allow food to get inside our body.

1. Inner wall
2. Outer wall
3. Organ between the inner and outer walls

In this intestinal organ, some portions are the constitute
components. They are (1) oil-like portion and (2) water-like
portion component. These components exist in the intestinal
organ, beginning from inner wall, then across the membrane
between two walls, then to outer walls, and then also beyond
the outer wall. Out of the outer wall, it is already inside the
human body.

Because of these constituent components present in the
intestinal wall, thus it allows and lets this treated food to get
into the inside of the human body. Why?

The food, after being treated through all the steps mentioned
above, is broken down into the three different major
substance groups.

1. Oil-like substance group (soluble into the oil)
2. Water-like substance group (soluble into water)

3. Insoluble substance group (not soluble in either oil or water)

Substances from the insoluble group can't be dissolved in any condition. Thus, it would be excreted out as feces from our body.

However, for the food broken down as oil-like substances in this organ, the force from intestinal movement would keep pressing and also moving it in this organ. Surely, it would touch the inner wall of this organ.

For this reason, the oil-like portion constituting the inner wall of this organ will certainly get the chance to contact the food's oil-like substance group. After they touch each other, because both are oil-like (soluble into oil), both of them dissolve (melt) into each other as a unified unit.

Because of the moving force from intestinal movement, this oil-like substance can flow in this oil-soluble channel, then across the member between the walls, then reach the outer wall of the intestinal organ. Finally, it will be released from the outer wall of the intestinal organ to get inside our body, and it is also when it gets into the bloodstream.

Now we understand how an oil-like substance can get inside our body.

For the remaining one, the water-like substance group, the process is similar to the principle and mechanism as the oil-like group substance. But the oil-like component is replaced by water-like component in the same intestinal organ.

Thus, the water-like substance group will also have a chance to touch and contact with the water-like component on this organ. Certainly, after they touch each other, both of them will also dissolve (melt) together into a unified unit. Thus, water-like group substance can also swim and flow into this water-soluble channel among the inner and outer walls across the member between the inner and outer walls of this organ.

Finally, this smaller-sized, water-like food substance group also will be released from the outer wall of the intestinal organ and then to the bloodstream.

Thus, they all now get inside the human body. Even if it is inside our body, how can they reach every organ and every tissue everywhere in our body?

The heart is the major part and organ to let those smaller pieces of food be able to enter everywhere in our body. This will be explained later. Without the heart, we cannot perform our daily human life. As mentioned above, it would not be possible for an excessive amount of food in our body to introduce the disease occurrence in our body. Thus, disease also happens from and is related to the heart's function.

Because digested food is already in its smallest size, they are now in the bloodstream. They will flow and move together with blood through the blood vessels as the blood circulates in our whole body everywhere, at every angle.

Now another question is, how can the blood be circulated in our body? Without circulation, the blood can't reach every part in our body.

What is the function of the heart in blood circulation?

The heart does the function of the heartbeat for blood circulation. It does this throughout our life until we die.

The function of the heartbeat is very simple, with two different actions there together.

1. Pumping (constriction)
2. Release (relaxation)

If there is only a pumping (constriction) action, no relaxation occurs in the heart, certainly, there is no heartbeat in the heart. We can't survive.

Vice versa, if there is only a relaxation action performed, no pumping is involved in the heart. Thus, there is also no heartbeat, and as a result, we don't survive.

For human survival, the heart must have a heartbeat function (pumping and relaxation together) to stay alive. Thus, the heartbeat action must be present there in humans for their whole lives.

As I understand from the medical society, the heartbeat occurs from central nerve triggers and controls. It also means that the heartbeat is directly related to the central nerve there. So far, we all know that this is the reason.

However, I have worked with the pharmaceutical industry for thirty years until I retired. During that working period, I sometimes went to the pharmacology department and watched them perform experiments. I found that some unexpected phenomenon happened in their experiment. At that time, I didn't pay attention at all.

Now I think this unexpected phenomenon is very important to what happens with the heartbeat.

In performing the experiments, the animal's heart was cut and removed and put into an incubator. The heart is no longer connected to the animal's body and also not connected with its central nerve system anymore. Unbelievably, in this situation, the heart was still jumping, and the heartbeat was there even for seven to eight hours. The heartbeat there occurred without the central nerve connection to the heart. Therefore, it is no reason for us to believe the explanation that the central nerve triggers and controls the heart (resulting in a heartbeat) is still true and valid.

Thus, I believe the relationship of the heartbeat to the heart has nothing to do with the central nerve.

Then how can the heart get the heartbeat function?

For heartbeat, we first have to be aware that the blood fills the heart in fully and is also in the entire network of blood vessels including the aorta and the veins. Then later on, the heart constricts. At the moment of constriction, the heart is required to have the force to trigger and push the blood out from the heart into the blood vessels. After that, all the force and energy are used up and gone by this pushing. No more energy is left over and available in the heart anymore. Pushing is the required force and energy in the heart. Thus, without this force in the heart, it definitely can't perform this pushing job.

After pushing, the amount of blood filling the heart is pushed out from it, and the pressure and force originally in the heart are also all gone. Thus, the space in the heart originally filled with blood is now empty and thus becomes a vacuum. In this empty space in the heart, there is no pressure; a low-pressure situation happens there.

However, after pushing, the more blood enters from the heart to the blood vessel. The amount of blood in the entire vessel is increased than without the pushing condition. Because the entire blood vessel—big or small, long or short—remained the same with no change, and the circulatory system is fully sealed. Therefore, the total blood pressure in the vessels would certainly change to higher, but the pressure in the heart after pushing is all gone; there is no more blood there, and the space is empty. Thus, in the heart there is no pressure or it is a low-pressure site. The blood vessels are high-pressure sites. Theoretically, the amount of blood would move and enter from a high-pressure site into the low-pressure site. The high-pressure site is the blood vessel. The low-pressure site is the heart. Thus, blood is then made from blood vessels, entering the low-blood pressure site, which is the heart. After blood enters, the heart is fully filled with blood until both sites reach a balance in pressure.

After both sites reach balance and blood fully fills the heart, the heart then is required for the next pushing, and the force is certainly required for the heart again. But the force or energy was already used up and gone and no longer there from the previous pushing. This force is now required for pushing, and at this moment, it is produced from a natural recharged and regenerated process in the heart. The heart itself acts as a rechargeable battery. The battery recharges from the source of the electrical current. This process of energy recharging the heart is done with the help of oxygen. The oxygen and air are brought into the heart by the blood from the lungs.

Oxygen is the energy source and acts as an electric current. The force is used after the previous push; oxygen and energy are also all used up, and there is no more force in the heart. Force and energy must be recharged to regenerate the force for pushing.

The heart, after pushing, then lets fresh blood enter the heart. The fresh blood enters the heart fully loaded with oxygen, which is carried from the lungs. Thus, oxygen is in the heart, and the heart can use it to recharge the force with this fresh blood. After the force and energy are recharged, a force is there already; the next push would also be available. The heartbeat starts again. This heartbeat cycle keep repeating. The heartbeat function occurs forever in our life. This is the mechanism of how the heartbeat occurs.

Pumping: what is pumping?

During the pumping step, the blood in the heart is completely pushed out by a force from the heart into the blood vessels. This force also allows the blood to flow into the blood vessels. Thus, this force is not only pushing the blood out from the heart but is also a force allowing the blood to move and flow in the blood vessels. Because of this force applied on the heart, the blood can thus flow to an initial limited distance in the blood vessels.

Release (relaxing): what is release?

After the pumping, the step of release (relaxing) follows. The amount of blood being pushed out in the step from pumping (pushing) now is ready for its return to the heart. After the blood returns, the heart now is fully filled with it and is also ready for the next pumping.

The heart, already filled with blood, is ready for next pumping action. The second pumping will also allow blood to move a farther distance.

These pumping and releasing actions keep going on in our life, and it is forever for our life until we die. Thus, blood will certainly circulate through our whole body and reach every part, everywhere, all the time in our life.

The digested food in the bloodstream will certainly circulate together with the blood and also reach everywhere, every organ and tissue in our body. Then it is also able to supply to every organ, every tissue, and every part in our body to use for maintaining their corresponding behavior daily. And the situation of an abnormal eating habit also affects this here. Then all the diseases occurring are directly or indirectly related to the heart's function. Without a heart, our life and physiological functions can't occur.

Therefore, the heart is the most important organ in the human body.

When talking about the occurrence of disease, we must always remember and remind ourselves that the heart should be considered in the discussion.

Now we should begin to talk about diseases.

Chapter 3

Hypertension

Hypertension would be discussed here but not in full detail because it has been already written in the book *The Mystery of Hypertension* published in 2009 (Cheung, 2009). It is also written in a Chinese version, 解開高血壓之謎, published in Taiwan, also in 2009 (張洪聲 2009).

Hypertension is directly related to the heart. Without the heart, there is no hypertension. No blood pressure can be found.

There are two different blood pressures.

1. *Systolic pressure* (Cheung, 2009)

   Systolic blood pressure results from contraction of the heart. During the contraction phase, the blood is forced into the blood vessels. It is from the heart in the constriction situation. In the constriction situation, after the heart constricts, all blood should be pushed out into the blood vessels. This pressure from heart constriction results in pushing all the blood out from heart to the blood vessel. Thus it also enables the blood flowing in the blood vessels. This force (constrictive force) is named systolic pressure (the higher value of the blood pressures, the top pressure value). Systolic pressure is, thus, also a pressure that results from the flow of blood through the blood vessels. Now for easy understanding, systolic pressure is the pressure that enables blood to move in the blood vessels. It also means that systolic pressure is the force (pressure) triggering the push of the blood moving in the blood vessels.

Blood flowing quickly or slowly in the vessels is strictly dependent on the diameter of the vessel's opening, big or small. The bigger the size, the faster the flow rate; the blood pressure is decreased or normal. Vice versa, the smaller the size, the slower the flow rate; the blood pressure is increased or high.

The bigger the size, the faster the movement of blood. Blood flows easier. Thus it requires less energy (pressure) to make the blood move.

A smaller size in the blood vessel makes the blood move slower. The reason is that when the diameter of the blood vessel's opening is smaller, the resistance for moving blood is higher and increased. Thus it requires more force to enable blood to move. This higher (increased) resistance thus causes blood to flow slowly along the vessels and also contributes to the higher blood pressure in our body. This higher blood pressure enables the blood to have a better flow and circulation in our body.

This higher blood pressure, in this case, is referred to as the high systolic pressure. Thus, we will have higher systolic pressure and higher blood pressure (hypertension). So blood *moving slowly* in the vessel results in higher blood pressure (high systolic pressure) occurring in our body.

The normal systolic pressure value is about *118-128*.

2. *Diastolic pressure* (Cheung, 2009)

Diastolic pressure occurs when the heart starts its relaxation cycle after it constricts. Thus, it will allow all the blood that had been pushed out from heart in the constriction cycle to return and fill the heart in the relaxation cycle.

This full amount of blood in the heart occupies volume and weight. This volume and weight from the amount of blood that returns to the heart press on it. The heart surely feels heavy with the weight applied on it; thus, it results in a pressure present in the heart. This pressure is referred to as diastolic pressure (the lower pressure value, the bottom pressure value).

The volume and weight of blood in the heart trigger this pressure. This is the heart's natural pressure and also is a basic and control blood pressures. We don't need to do anything as long as that much amount of blood is in the heart. That value of blood pressure is automatically natural there. This pressure value is directly related to the amount of blood present in the heart. It is also the pressure that allows the heart to hold blood.

Thus, *more* blood in the heart results in having a higher blood pressure. It is a higher diastolic pressure.

The normal diastolic pressure value is *68-78*.

No matter which blood pressure—either systolic or diastolic or both—is high, it will result in hypertension occurring in us.

Therefore, why are the blood pressures higher in us? Now it is clear to us. It is from the situation where the blood either moves slowly in the blood vessels or an increased amount of blood is found in the heart.

Those symptoms are the major reasons causing a higher blood pressure in us. However, there is also another situation resulting in a higher blood pressure. For the time being, the other reason is not talked about here. We will discuss it later.

Now we talk about why higher blood pressures are occurring from either case.

A. Blood moves slowly in the heart vessel

It has been already discussed. It is because of the size of a blood vessel's opening is smaller. We can't touch the vessels inside our body. How can its size change to become smaller?

The reason is strictly from the vessel being compressed by a constrictor agent, angiotensin II (Cheung, 2003/2009). This constrictor is produced in our body by the angiotensin-converting enzyme, ACE (Cheung, 2003/2009). From now on, for easy understanding, we change the word *enzyme* to *machine* (Cheung, 2009). The machine makes the constrictor produced in our body, thus leading to the constricting action in our body. This results in constricting the size of blood vessels such that they are smaller afterward.

This constriction, *vasoconstriction* (Cheung, 2003/2009), is the major cause resulting in the size of vessels' openings being smaller then also leading to a higher systolic pressure in our body. After constriction, the size of a blood vessel opening is smaller. The blood vessel itself thus becomes much harder than it used to be.

If the size of the blood vessel's opening is smaller, the resistance for the blood flowing through it is higher. Certainly, its blood flow is slowed down. This results in a higher blood pressure.

B. When more blood is in the heart, the reason is from the intake of more salt/sodium chloride (Cheung, 2009)

Western and Chinese doctors all know that. So they always warn the patient to take less salt in their diet to avoid absorbing increased amounts of water into the body. Therefore more blood in the body requires absorbing more water into the body. Certainly, it requires taking more salt in the body first. Salt thus acts as an intermediate to introduce more water into the blood then also into the heart. Thus, more water in the blood certainly results in increased amount of blood in the heart.

An increase (amount or volume) of blood in the heart also contributes the property of its weight. Thus, for an increased amount of blood in the heart, the weight of blood is heavier for the heart to hold. It thus exerts a higher pressure on the heart. This higher blood pressure is a higher diastolic pressure (the lower blood pressure value, the bottom pressure value).

This diastolic pressure is the pressure and force that apply to holding those amounts of blood in the heart. Without this pressure, those amounts of blood are possibly not there in the heart.

At this moment, we understand that both situations of increased blood amount and decreased blood flow will result in a situation of high blood pressure (either one or both systolic and diastolic).

Other reasons can cause higher blood pressure. Now, it can be discussed here.

1. Faster heart rate (Cheung, 2009)
2. Increased amount of cholesterol present in the body (Cheung, 2009)

Both these situations are not related to the situations mentioned above.

Now the other reasons are as follow:

1. Faster heart rate

    If the heart's pumping rate is faster, it may likely result in a higher blood pressure. The speed of the heart pumping can change to either slow or fast based on the situation. This is a natural phenomenon in the human body. It is from actions or also from a change in emotions in our body, such as thinking, talking, running, being angry, doing backyard work, or doing heavy jobs and so on. After doing all these, your heart's pumping speed will be much faster than before. The blood pressure will automatically be much higher too.

    To learn why a faster pumping rate results in a higher blood pressure, please refer to the book *The Mystery of Hypertension* by Hong Son Cheung (2009).

2. Increased amount of cholesterol

An increased amount of cholesterol will result in the situation of higher blood pressure. Cholesterol is a heavy, sticky material or compound. Its presence will result in cholesterol adhering to the vessel firmly. Then, it will fill in the space of this vessel. The opening in this vessel becomes smaller and smaller. This smaller space is a result of cholesterol filling the opening. Cholesterol has also been recognized to result in the situation of a harder blood vessel.

Because the size of the vessel becomes smaller, the ability of blood to flow or move in this vessel surely becomes much less and slows down quite a bit. Therefore, because the blood moves slowly, the systolic blood pressure is also higher.

Higher systolic pressure is also here, but certainly, it is from the situation of the cholesterol filling in the space of the vessel. And it is not from the case of the blood vessel being constricted.

Even medical society and physicians mention that the situation of blood vessels becoming harder (vasoconstriction) is from the plaque building up and the cholesterol filling in the vessels.

Truly, in this case, the blood vessel itself remains as soft as it was originally (the blood vessels themselves remaining at the same flexibility without any difference). When it becomes harder, it is from a vessel wall built up with cholesterol. For the blood vessel itself, it still has the same softness and flexibility as it did originally.

Now, we understand why higher blood pressure is occurring to us.

But even though we understand why blood pressure occurs, we have no idea what kind of food or diet triggers the higher blood pressure.

As mentioned above, in the medical society, Chinese and Western physicians are aware that a high blood pressure occurs from taking too much salt in our diet. Thus, salt is considered as a dietary reason of high blood pressure.

Even if it is, however, it is still not clear to us why salt would cause a higher blood pressure. We already know that the salt absorbs water and, thus, results in a high blood pressure.

Salts. There are many kinds of salt in our diet. Sodium salt, chloride salt, and especially sodium chloride salt (Cheung, 2009) are the most important sources contributing to a high blood pressure in our body. Sodium salt and chloride salt (Cheung, 2009) are different salts from each other, but they are single salt and a single compound. Sodium chloride salt is sodium and chloride combined together as another new single salt. This one is the major salt in our diet that causes our high blood pressure.

The reason salt is known to increase blood pressure is that it makes our body absorb more water. This kind of salt is *generally* referred to as sodium chloride. It is true. Sodium chloride salt has a strong ability to absorb water.

Unfortunately, this hypertension just indicates that blood pressure is increasing (high blood pressure). But which blood pressure is higher, systolic or diastolic? Thus, it is still an unclear question to us regarding hypertension.

Even the role of sodium chloride in contributing to the property of absorbing water is known. This information is supplied from the field of chemistry. However, using this property in the medical field is not totally correct. Therefore, it leads us to the wrong direction to understand hypertension.

The ability of sodium chloride salt to absorb water is not from the sodium chloride salt (Cheung, 2009). Sodium chloride salt contains two parts: sodium and chloride. Sodium and chloride are different from each other. The part of sodium is the one that contributes this ability to absorb water. Therefore, because sodium is part of sodium chloride, sodium provides this ability to absorb water; certainly, sodium chloride also contributes this ability to absorb water. Thus, it is clear that the ability of absorbing water is not from sodium chloride; it is from sodium only (Cheung, 2009).

It had been mentioned above that more blood in the heart would result in a higher blood pressure. More blood in the heart certainly results in a higher blood pressure. It is a higher diastolic pressure (Cheung, 2009).

Thus, sodium absorbs more water into our body. An increased amount of water is in our body.

Why does it cause an increased diastolic blood pressure?

The question is, if higher blood pressure is from absorbing increased amounts of water into our body, then why is a higher pressure only found in the blood and not somewhere else in our body? It does not make any sense at all.

To make sense of this, to answer this question, it must be modified as follows.

Sodium chloride salt absorbs more water into our body. More water is in our body; the heart is part of our body. What thing or material is in the heart? No question, it is blood in the heart. Blood is a combination of liquid materials. The most important component in blood is water.

More water is absorbed into our body. Certainly, the increased amount of water will also automatically enter the heart. The increased amount of water entering the heart surely results in the water amount also increasing in the heart. Naturally, the higher water amount in the heart, the higher amount of blood in the heart there is, theoretically. The amount of blood is increased in the heart. Naturally, the diastolic blood pressure is also increased.

The increased amount of blood in the heart (more water absorbed from sodium intake) results in the occurrence of hypertension (higher diastolic pressure) happening.

Now the situation that more water is absorbed into our body from sodium intake is clear to us. The higher blood pressure is the diastolic pressure only.

After this, we may conclude, salt—not only sodium chloride salt, but the other sodium salts also—has this property to absorb water. Thus, it can happen from any kind of salt as long as that salt contains sodium.

Therefore, all sodium salts (Cheung, 2009) will contribute this property of water absorption, such as sodium glutamate. Sodium glutamate is also branded as Ac'cent. It is used in cooking, especially in Chinese cuisine, to make food taste better. However, Ac'cent also contains sodium (sodium ion). Therefore, sodium is in Ac'cent and can be a reason why after eating from a Chinese restaurant, we feel thirsty and drink lots of water.

Now we know the reason for the high diastolic blood pressure in human body. The sodium diet is a main reason why the diastolic pressure is high.

However, which diet can cause a higher systolic blood pressure is still unknown. We only know that from above, high systolic pressure is from the constrictor (angiotensin II) produced in our body constricting a blood vessel smaller and then harder. The size (diameter) of the blood vessel opening is smaller, and blood flow and movement are slowed down, thus resulting in the increased high systolic pressure.

The diet that causes high systolic blood pressure is still waiting to be discovered.

Sodium, as already mentioned, is a dietary agent that triggers a high diastolic pressure, but whether it affects high systolic pressure is never mentioned. Is it also from sodium?

From the facts and from experiments and studies known, sodium is not a dietary agent that causes high systolic pressure (Cheung, 2009).

We already mentioned that a high systolic pressure occurs because of the constrictor produced in the body. The constrictor produced in the body requires a human machine (named angiotensin-converting enzyme, ACE) there (Cheung, 2003/2009).

For the machine to make this product, it requires natural electric energy to do its work and function. Without electricity there, the machine can't function to do the work to make the product.

For the machine (human machine, ACE) to do the work to produce constrictors in the body, it also requires *some source of electric energy* in the body. This electricity is from our dietary agents.

This electricity from the diet is not surprising at all. It is chloride (Cheung, 2009; Cushman, et al., 1971). And it is required by the machine (ACE) to function to produce constrictors. It comes from the sodium chloride salt. Again sodium chloride contains the chloride part. Chloride provides an electric current for this machine to produce constrictors. Therefore, the sodium chloride will also contribute this identical function or property as chloride for the machine. But it must be emphasized again that this function is from chloride itself alone.

Chloride is used as electricity for the machine to produce constrictors. The blood vessel will thus be constricted further resulting in the smaller diameter of the blood vessel's opening. Blood flowing or moving in this smaller opening vessel must be slowed down; the blood pressure (systolic pressure), thus, is raised higher.

Of course, besides the sodium chloride salt, other chloride salts (such as potassium chloride, ferrous chloride, and so on) all contain chloride parts. Thus, these kinds of salts in our body will also contribute to the higher systolic pressure in our body.

Thus, we can conclude that sodium chloride salt is really the one single substance in our body that can trigger higher blood pressures. It is also the cause for both systolic and diastolic pressures being simultaneously higher in our body (Cheung, 2009). No other one can do it.

Therefore, we also understand that if in case any kind of sodium salt and any kind of chloride salt are both present in our body, both the systolic and diastolic pressures will certainly rise higher together in our body. This function is just the same as when the single salt sodium chloride alone is present there in our body; there is no difference (Cheung, 2009).

Therefore, if we want to make sure our systolic and diastolic blood pressures are both at normal values, the amount of salt intake—especially sodium chloride salt—must be adjusted and should be monitored daily using the blood pressure measurement gauge to be sure.

If the pressure is high, the diet's salt intake amount must be cut down; if it is the opposite, increase the amount. This should be done and verified daily.

We must remember that even if we are aware of this situation and have also already taken little amounts of salt from the diet, most of us sometimes still find our blood pressures are high and cannot be reduced to the normal pressure values.

The reason the pressure is still high even if the amount of salt taken is very little for us is usually from the thinking and guessing. In fact, it is not at all; the salt amount is still possibly high. Our body will let us know whether the salt amount is still high or low. It is from measuring pressures, checking the high or low values obtained.

The other reason is, some humans may be so sensitive to the salt amount there even if it is low. Thus, monitor your blood pressure daily to control your salt intake; it is a very important step to do for us to follow control of the salt amount. Doing this step can help us avoid making those missed judgments, guesses, and suspicions.

Chapter 4

Heart Attack

Hypertension will seriously result in a heart attack. It is well-known by humans and also known in the medical society. Thus, Western and Chinese doctors are also aware of this. Therefore lowering your blood pressure to the normal value is a perfect approach to avoid a heart attack.

In a way, this is true, but it is not totally correct.

Hypertension from the dietary agent sodium chloride causes (1) chloride to trigger the openings of blood vessels to become smaller, resulting in a higher systolic pressure, and (2) sodium to trigger too much water absorption, resulting in too much blood in the heart and, thus, a high diastolic pressure.

Practically, these kinds of hypertension will not have the chance to cause a heart attack.

Why? Because the blood pressures are higher.

1. Systolic higher pressure (from this phenomenon)

    If the blood vessels are constricted, the opening size of the vessel is certainly smaller. The blood movement in the vessel is slowed down, thus resulting in hypertension (high systolic pressure).

From this phenomenon, the blood moving is slower but can still move freely. The blood vessel becomes narrow, but the vessel is *never sealed and closed* completely. For this reason, under this condition—from this kind of hypertension and from this high systolic pressure—a heart attack surely has no chance of happening.

2. Diastolic higher pressure (from this phenomenon)

It is because of an increased amount of blood in the heart, thus resulting to the hypertension (higher diastolic pressure) in our body.

For this reason—an *increased amount of blood* in the heart—the blood is certainly overloaded in the heart. The heart must work much harder than usual. Certainly, it is not good for the heart at all. It definitely *results in a disease of the heart.* Usually, it is a heart disease but not the heart attack. *A heart disease and a heart attack are not the same.* Thus, a heart attack, therefore, certainly should not and never be from hypertension (high diastolic pressure). From the aforementioned, the higher blood pressure (hypertension including both systolic and diastolic pressures) surely has no possible chance resulting in the occurrence of a heart attack.

What causes a heart attack?

It is from a *high level of cholesterol presence* in the blood circulating system.

Cholesterol is a soft, *solid*, adhesive, and waxy compound (a kind similar to oil, a lipid component compound). Solids can't be moved; thus, it is not flowing by itself at all in the blood vessel. But it can be moved and flows together with the blood by the push of the moving blood. In case there is a large amount of oily substances (fat, oil, and cholesterol) present, they accumulate in the blood circulation system such as the blood vessels, aorta, and so on. Cholesterol might be sticky and adhesive there. Then it will block the partial opening of vessels or tubelike organs and prevent the flow of blood in the system.

It is also known that cholesterol is not soluble in the water and also insoluble in blood. Thus, water and blood cannot dissolve the cholesterol to make it into a liquid form for flowing in the system.

In the circulatory system, this situation contributes two different symptoms in our body.

1. The serious one, where cholesterol that accumulates in the vessels, aorta, or others is too much. The opening pathways in *the vessels become very narrow and, possibly, is even completely closed and sealed.* Thus, the blood flowing there certainly is very slow or even completely stopped. It may result in the following:

    In the blood circulation, if *blood moves slowly or completely stops, the oxygen brought* by the blood to the heart *is either too small an amount or even not enough.* Thus, an *oxygen deficiency situation* occurs in the heart. This occurrence must result from the case in that vessel in the nearly sealed or completely closed situation. This vessel especially is the one that directly lets the blood flow into the heart. When the vessels are sealed, surely, there is no blood flowing in, resulting to *no energy or force* that will sustain the heartbeat, **and this may lead to a heart attack.**

2. The next situation is if the cholesterol amount is not too much and is not that serious. Certainly, cholesterol accumulating in the vessel is also not that bad, and the vessel is never sealed completely. The opening space is surely not that narrow. The blood is still able to move freely, but it is slower.

    Even though the blood is still moving slowly, the oxygen deficiency is certainly not in the heart. Therefore, the heart attack will not likely happen in this situation from this amount of cholesterol. However, a heart attack happens even if it does not occur in this circumstance; instead, hypertension (higher blood pressure) is the result here.

    The heart attack is not from the hypertension but rather might be from the *large amount of cholesterol* present in the blood vessels. Thus, it also blocks most of or completely shuts down the blood's movement in the circulation system. Then, it triggers an oxygen (energy) deficiency in the heart. The heart attack thus occurs.

    Therefore, if cholesterol is present, and if the *amount* is not *too much or too serious*, it contributes to a different symptom; hypertension occurs. This hypertension is triggered from cholesterol, and it certainly does not have the chance to cause a heart attack.

Now it is clear to us that a heart attack is not from hypertension. A heart attack occurs from a large amount of cholesterol being present and blocking the blood flowing into the heart.

Thus, a case of oxygen and energy deficiency is occurring in the heart, which can then result in a heart attack occurring.

Thus, no matter if hypertension occurs from the intake of a high-salt (sodium chloride) diet or from a certain amount of cholesterol stuck on the vessel wall, a heart attack will not likely occur from hypertension.

This is the next item we talk about.

Chapter 5

Stroke

Western and Chinese doctors are also aware that hypertension will trigger a stroke.

Look at the air balloon: if we blow air into the balloon, there is air pressure in the balloon. In case we blow too much air into the balloon, the air pressure in the balloon is high. If it is too high, the balloon is not able to resist this high pressure. Thus, the balloon will explode and break a hole and let the air out from this broken location on the balloon.

On the other hand, we have blood pressure in our blood vessels. For the same reason, if the blood pressure is too high, the blood vessels are unable to resist this high pressure, and then the vessel also will explode with the wound as the hole. Thus, the wound also will allow blood to leak out from the vessel. If this vessel is in the brain, a stroke may occur.

We also know that if a stroke happens, it may result in having a part of the body paralyzed.

Question: why, after a stroke, is part of your body paralyzed and may you lose the ability to move around?

For instance, suppose we cut a hole in our body; blood will leak out from the wound. Sooner or later, the blood will coagulate and heal this wounded area. Then the blood will stop leaking out from the wound.

This high blood pressure situation can happen to any vessel in human body. That vessel may explode, and blood will also leak out from this wound.

In some cases, this blood vessel is in an area in the brain and near the area of the central nervous system. The central nervous system is very complicated and its size may not be too big; however, it controls many physiological functions related to behavior. Certainly, actions such as one's moving ability may also be controlled by this.

This part of the blood vessel, if the pressure is too high, will not be able to resist it, and thus, this vessel may explode and let blood leak out from this area. For the same reason, the blood sooner or later will coagulate and heal the vessel's wounded area in the brain.

The blood will coagulate there in the vessel's wound and the whole area. After blood coagulates there, the blood will not be able to pour out from the hole and from the wound anymore.

However, the area of the wound (hole) includes the wound itself (hole) and the opening channel of the same vessel (hole and internal vessel connecting to the hole) together as a whole unit. The opening channel (internal vessel only) is for the blood flowing in this vessel. The hole is for the blood leaking out only.

However, this whole wound unit is originally for the blood flowing. Our defense system and our body have no way to tell the difference between them. Which one is the wound (hole) area and which one is not and which one is the internal opening channel of blood vessel?

Thus, the defense system and body recognize them both as a wound area. Therefore, coagulation is not only on the wound (hole). The coagulation also happens inside the blood vessel connected to the hole. Thus, blood will coagulate at both spots. They are the whole area, the wound (hole) and blood vessel together.

Due to blood coagulating in both spots of the whole vessel, the blood is not leaking out from the wound (hole), but the blood has also stopped flowing into this same blood vessel.

The blood certainly can't be delivered anymore and any farther to the area beyond this coagulated (sealed and closed) position. Thus, the blood vessel beyond this sealed position cannot get blood supplies anymore. Only a limited amount of blood is still remaining in this area beyond this sealed position.

Blood carries oxygen (energy). Thus, only a limited amount of oxygen is still in this limited amount of blood there. After the cells in this vessel use up all this amount of oxygen, those cells in those vessel areas die. That is not the only situation. On the other hand, no blood and oxygen can be further supplied to the area beyond this coagulated position. Unfortunately, there is no chance for blood and oxygen supplying to them anymore from this sealed situation. Then, a stroke can occur.

Why, after a stroke, a part of the body may be paralyzed

To understand this—why after a stroke occurs, the body can't move anymore—know that actions such as moving can be performed in our body because it is connected to the nervous system. The central nervous system is the major part for operating those functions. The central nervous system will require sending a command (information, message) to tell which part of our body to do the action. For example, when it tells the arm to move, the central nervous system will send a command (information) to the arm and ask it to move around. After the arm receives this message (information), the arm moves immediately.

Therefore, this command (message or information) is the *original information* beginning from central nervous part. This command (information) is received by the arm; it is *receiving information* also present in the arm (another location). After the arm receives this information, it responds with a moving action in the arm immediately.

Now, this command (original and receiving information) is present in both locations—the central nervous system and the arm (original and another location) respectively. This same information is in two different locations, but they are still the same command (information) for proceeding with the same action.

Question: how can the same information exist in two different places in the human body?

To make us understand how this same information can be present in two different places in human body, we use a binocular as an example.

If we look at a thing or a person, we can see the image of that person. Looking through the binoculars, the person is still where it was originally, but an enlarged image of that person is displayed inside the binoculars.

Thus, using the binoculars, we can find two images for the same person there. The original one is still in that location. The other one is inside in the binoculars. Both images are there.

Even if it is the same image of that person there, looking through the binoculars, the image of that body truly exists in two different places (locations). Therefore, this phenomenon is just as the aforementioned. One is in the original place and *original image*. The other is inside the binoculars' lens, another image (*receiving image*). There are two images in this case too. The image is also in two different locations. In this phenomenon, the same image of that person is in two different locations, found at the original location and in the binoculars. It is just as in the case of the same command in two different parts (arm and central nervous system) in the human body. Both of them are in two different places; there is no difference.

For another example, imagine when we take a picture by using a camera. First we have to see that person's image in the camera and then click the button to take a picture of that person. After picture taking, the image of that person is not present only in the camera. Its image is also present and stored in the camera, on the film or memory chip. Thus, the image of that person is not only in the camera, but it is also in the film and the memory chip. It is also in two different locations and places. This phenomenon is exactly the same as the phenomenon occurring in the human body.

How can it be the same one image existing in two different places in both scenes using binoculars and cameras?

The image must be treated as a message, information, or signal here. The information (signal or message) can also be thought of as merchandise. It can be sent (delivered or transported) to a different location. The real merchandise (commercial product) can be shipped to another place, such as a store, by truck. However, after being shipped, this merchandise can only be in one place and is impossible to be present in both places.

Information can be treated as merchandise, but it is not real merchandise. Solid material (merchandise) is a real thing. After transporting, this real thing (solid thing) can't be present in two places.

Because information is not real merchandise, thus, after transportation, it (the information) must be in two or more different places (locations), and it certainly is not only in one place. It can be explained below.

The message, information, is not a thing or material. It cannot be held and grabbed by hand. Thus it can't be touched. The information—such as a word, letter, or image—is not really there. It is just information and a message because it is not really existent in our society and can't be touched, held, or grabbed. Thus, it is an unreal item, not existing there. Therefore, this information and message can only be transported by unreal vehicles. This vehicle here is energy.

What is information or message?

Information may be classified into three categories

1. By seeing
2. By hearing
3. By feeling

1. By seeing, a person is physically there and truly exists and can be touched, held, and grabbed by our hand. A person is a real thing. However, after seeing this person,

there is also an image of this person. This image can't be held and touched by hand. The original image (*original information*) of this person with this person's body is together as a unit, which can be seen with the eyes while the body can be held, touched, and grabbed by the hand.

Even the image of this person can be seen into the eyes. However, that person and its original image still remain at the same place, on the same spot, without moving. With our eyes, we can see that person; it is only an image of that person delivered into our eyes. It is not that person delivered to our eyes. And it is also not the same image from the original. It is a different image. This image seen in the eyes is a second and delivered image (*receiving information*), and it also can't be touched, held, and grabbed. The phenomenon of original image delivered the second image into our eyes. It is the occurrence of information (or message) transferred and transmitted to our eyes.

2. By hearing, music or sound can be heard from a source, such as a speaker, then this music information is sent to our ears. The speaker can be touched, held, and grabbed, but sound cannot. The sound and speaker are one whole unit; without either one there, sound certainly cannot be heard in our ears. Even when we can hear the sound in our ears, the original sound (*original information*) and source still remain in their original places (speaker); there is no change.

The sound we can hear in our ears, theoretically, is not the same original sound. It is already a different sound from the original. It is a delivered sound (delivered information). It may be considered a secondary sound (delivered sound, *receiving information*).

This sound heard is also the so-called information or message delivery.

3. By feeling, a temperature change is one of the natural environments proceeding. Temperature changes may happen naturally. It also can happen from a source such as a heater. A heater can be touched, held, and grabbed, but heat cannot.

   Without a source heater, the heat certainly can't be produced. Therefore, the heat and heater together are also one unit. Heat from a heater should be considered original heat (*original information*). The heat delivered to us is already not the same heat as the original. This heat delivered to us is a secondary heat (*delivered heat, received information*). This heat that reaches us is also called information or message transferring, transportation, and delivery.

To make it easy to understand, in the computer, there are several parts combined together as one computer unit. The monitor (screen), hard drive, keyboard, and mouse are part of one computer.

1. The monitor is the place (screen), the information, message, or data that can be seen on the computer.

2. The hard drive is the data storage center (vault) for the computer, storing all information and data, such as letters, pictures, videos, and all others.

3. The keyboard and mouse are a work center to command which part of the computer to function (do the work). It is such as what information should be *displayed on the screen* or what data (information) is being stored or transferred in or from the *hard drive*.

In case we want to get online (on a website) on the computer, after getting online, the website automatically displays on the computer screen.

Even if the website is displayed on the screen, the website itself (the carrier) is still located in its original site or place, never gone. For this phenomenon, the same website (information, message) not only exists and is present on the computer screen; it is also presented in its original website carrier. Therefore, it exists and is presented also in two different places or locations.

For another instance, if we want to write a letter, we must load the Microsoft Word file first from the hard drive (the storage center). After the Microsoft Word file is displayed on the screen, we can then write words and letters in this file. Later after finishing writing, this letter can be stored into the hard drive. After being stored, this letter is also displayed on the computer screen and present in the storage center. This same letter image not only exists and is present on the computer screen. It is also exists and is present in the storage center, and it is also in two different places.

However, even with this letter present in two different places, this letter can be stored from the computer screen into the storage center. It also can be transferred (sent) to the computer screen to display from the storage center. Thus, it can be transferred from each other without any problem.

Thus the data transfer on the computer also happened in two different places and locations. Even if it is in two different places, it is for the same data or information. However, the first one is the original one (*original information*); the other is the saved or delivered one (received information). Therefore, they still are different; truly, it is not the same one.

This information transfer also is happening in the computer. How can it be transferred to each other in the computer?

For this kind of transferring, the computer parts are connected by many electrical wires or cables together to one unit. These electrical wires and cables would function as the transportation or traffic *highway* for the information transfer or transportation from each part.

For information transporting, they are not real things and real products there. Thus, a real vehicle such as a truck can't transport them. *Information* here may look like a *product* and *merchandise*, but it is not a real product and merchandise.

Thus, information transporting must be by an unreal *vehicle*. *This unreal vehicle is an electric current*; thus, an electrical current (energy) is a vehicle, and it's transporting through the highway. This highway is the *electrical wire or cable*.

Computer is connected by many electrical wires and cables. To make the computer work, the computer must be turned on. After the computed is turned on, the electric current (*vehicle*) is running through the whole computer in those traffic *highways* of electric wires. Information transporting from each other in the computer thus proceeds to function by an electric current (unreal vehicle).

An electric current is energy. Energy and electric currents are also invisible. It is also not a real thing or vehicle in our society. But energy and currents are the vehicles for information transfer. Thus, these energy and electric currents are not even visible. It is able to transport those unreal issues (*merchandise*). Those issues are also invisible, unable to be held, touched, and grabbed (such as information, messages, and data) in the computer.

Now, we understand that information, messages, and data can be transported and transferred to each other in the computer. It is because of the energy (vehicle) there in the electrical wire (highway).

There are cases when the power of the computer is shut down or that the connecting cable is disconnected. Thus, there is no energy in the cable. If there is no energy (vehicle), the information certainly can't be transferred to each other. The computer will not be able to function anymore, and we may also call or refer to it as a computer "stroke."

This computer symptom is because there is no energy or electric current (vehicle) there in the electrical wire (highway). Thus, to make sure the computer is in working condition, those wires must be connecting to each other. The electrical power also should be turned on.

The information and message thus can be transported and transferred in the computer. Computer stroke certainly is not there.

Now it is clear to us that *information* can be transported, but it only occurs in the case when energy (vehicle) is there.

As discussed above, the central nervous system requires the oxygen (energy) supplied to them. It is no longer available.

Oxygen is energy; it is also a vehicle. With no oxygen, no vehicle is there. Information transferred certainly can't function anymore, and information can't be delivered to where it is supposed to reach, such as an arm.

Therefore, the arm receives no information. The arm certainly cannot respond to a moving action. If there is no moving action in the arm, the arm, thus is paralyzed. If this situation occurs to half our body permanently, certainly, half of our body is paralyzed.

Thus, how can we be so sure that energy also is the one and is the reason? Is it also playing this role in our human body, resulting in a stroke?

How can we prove this point?

For the computer

In a computer, we can disconnect the power to shut down the computer or part of it to prove the point. However, with energy in our body, we have no way to disconnect it. Thus, how can we prove that is true? That is the real reason to us. The stroke and the half-body paralysis—are they truly from this reason of lack of energy?

For human body

We cannot even disconnect and shut down the energy in our body; we can try to reduce the heat's amount from the source to prove this point. For a reduced heat, the energy may be insufficient. It is just as to turn off the power situation. There is no difference.

Suppose in the wintertime, in some zones, the temperature can drop very low, such as 20° to 30° Fahrenheit (F) or-6.6 to-1.1° centigrade (C). The room temperature, however, can be set up to a suitable temperature such as 70° F (21.1°C) to make us feel comfortable.

However, to save for the heating bill, if the room temps are reduced or dropped to between 40°-50° F or (4.4°-10° C), our whole body will feel very cold. After being in this environment too long, our hands will feel the loss of its original flexibility. The feeling is terrible; the hand is numb. The ability of the hands to hold or pick up things cannot be performed as well as usual. This is because the heat supply is reduced and dropped resulting in it. Thus numbness is the symptom of partial paralysis or minor stroke situation in our body.

From this phenomenon of numbness, it is no question that energy is the reason that plays a role in our human body for transferring messages. If there is no energy or less energy, or no blood or less blood there, information and commands certainly cannot be delivered and transferred normally from central nervous system to half of our body. Stroke and numbness thus can occur.

Energy for transferring can be from three different cases. In the first one, the amount of blood and oxygen is fully supplied, and the blood flowing rate (speeding) is at normal. In the second one, the blood and oxygen amount is either fully or not enough there, but the rate (speed) for transferring surely is at reduced or much slowing situation. In the third one, no more blood and oxygen are supplied, and no transferring can be performed.

In the first situation, information transferring is normal. There are no stroke and numbness. Functions are normal in our life.

If it is in the second situation, the rate for the information transfer is slowed down a lot. Thus, numbness (partial paralysis) occurs.

If it is in the third case, no information can be transferred at all from each other. A stroke will result.

If a stroke from higher blood pressure occurs, the symptom of blood coagulation certainly also occurs.

In this situation, if the time of the stroke is not too long, you could take a blood-thinner drug such as Coumadin to prevent your stroke from occurring. The anticoagulant drug Coumadin can make your blood thinner and prevent blood coagulation from occurring in the vessel and wound area. Thus, the blood can continue moving in the vessel. Oxygen (vehicle) is always there to be supplied to the central nervous system. Information transferring can be continuous. Thus, a stroke can be avoided.

However, this is not the only reason to have a stroke. There is another reason to cause a stroke. It is not from a higher blood pressure that causes the blood vessel to burst a hole and get a wound. There is also no blood coagulation resulting from this stroke.

It is from the large dose of cholesterol in the body. An overdose (excess amount) of cholesterol in our body will clog up the open spaces of blood vessels. If the amount is too high there, the open space may be completely blocked and fully sealed. Thus, no blood can move and flow beyond this sealed position. No oxygen is there too. If this blood vessel is in the brain and it is also the same vessel as in the hypertension situation, then there is no difference, and the stroke will certainly be there from this condition of cholesterol-blocked blood vessels.

Stroke happens if the blood vessels are clogged by cholesterol and sealed as a result. The blood-thinner drug is useless for this kind of stroke.

Now it is clear to us that a stroke can happen from these two situations:

1. Hypertension
2. An overdose of cholesterol in the body blocked and sealed a vessel

Either one could result in a stroke.

Now we understand that cholesterol is very important to us.

However, generally we know two kinds of important cholesterols.

1. Good cholesterol, HDL (high-density lipoprotein)
2. Bad cholesterol, LDL (low-density lipoprotein)

Why is HDL good cholesterol and LDL bad cholesterol?

Generally speaking, HDL is good cholesterol because it doesn't cause the diseases of heart attack and stroke. LDL is different; it can cause diseases of heart attack and stroke in us. Thus, LDL is bad cholesterol.

Why doesn't HDL, or good cholesterol, cause diseases of heart attack and stroke in humans? And why does LDL give us heart attacks and strokes?

HDL (good cholesterol) and LDL (bad cholesterol) are both cholesterols. Even if both of them are cholesterols, they have different structures. Because of these differences, each of them displays its own special property and ability to maintain their different symptoms in the human body.

The property of LDL

LDL (low-density lipoprotein) is a soft, sticky white solid. Because it is a solid, it can't move by itself in any circumstance. But it can move and flow only by the force of pushing, such as from liquid or blood flowing in the vessels. Certainly, it could be moved away by blood pushing in the bloodstream during the blood circulation.

The sticky LDL adheres on the blood vessels. In the beginning, there will be no plaque built up there. The size of the vessel opening for the blood flowing thus remains the same.

However, blood continuously circulates in the vessels and never stops in our life. In the beginning, LDL is pushed away from the vessel by flowing blood; no plaque builds up there. However, blood and LDL stay in the circulatory system and make contact with the inner wall of the blood vessels. Then sooner or later, LDL will have the chance to stick on the inner walls of the vessels.

Plaque thus begins to build up in a vessel. Later on, more and more LDL will continuously stick together on this area with plaque. The plaque thus becomes bigger and bigger. The opening for the blood flow and circulation in the blood vessel is certainly smaller and smaller. Blood circulation becomes harder and harder. The heart thus will do much more heavy work to make blood flow. A heart attack or stroke will happen sooner or later because of this.

Thus, LDL is classified as bad cholesterol.

The property of HDL

HDL is not a solid material and compound. It may be more like thick liquid. A solid can't flow by itself in the vessels and tubes. A liquid can move and flow in the vessels and tubes by itself.

HDL is a thick liquid. A liquid can flow in the vessels. HDL also doesn't have a sticky and adhesive ability to build up the plaque in the vessel. Thus the HDL can move and flow freely in the vessel together with blood. Since no plaque can't build up in the blood vessels, heart attacks and strokes certainly can't result from HDL in us. This is the reason HDL is good cholesterol.

Besides that, there is another important reason there. Cholesterol is an oily component; thus, its behavior is similar to the functions of oil-like substances. HDL and LDL are both cholesterols; thus, both of them are oil-like substances.

Initially, LDL is a very small and tiny particle in the blood vessel. Even LDL can be adhered to the vessel, but not tightly enough in the beginning.

However, blood is always circulating in the blood vessel. HDL, if it is also present with the blood, will also flow together with the blood. As blood circulates in the blood vessels, it certainly will contact the surface of the inner vessel walls. The sticky or adhesive LDL forms plaque there on the walls of the vessel. Certainly, it will also have the chance to contact with the circulating blood and HDL.

After contact, first, the force of blood flowing also tries to push the adhesive LDL away from the surface of the blood vessel to remove this plaque. In case, it can't be pushed away by the blood flow's force.

Following this, the HDL also contacts this plaque of LDL. Because both HDL and LDL are oil-like substances, both of them, after touching, can be dissolved into each other as one liquid form. LDL dissolves and merges together with HDL as a liquid; thus, LDL plaque can flow and move away from the surface of the vessel together with HDL and the blood. Thus, the built-up LDL plaque disappears from that spot on the blood vessel.

The plaque is gone—no more LDL sticking on the blood vessel. Thus, the blood can flow easily and freely in circulation. This is the reason why HDL is good cholesterol. Therefore, the more amount of HDL in the body, the better it is for us

Chapter 6

Diabetes

A lot of people are interested in the subject of diabetes. Most of them are aware of it and also know what it is about.

Diabetes is a disease. As mentioned above, all diseases may occur from eating. Usually, it is the amount of that food or diet changing from normal (suitable) to an increased amount in our body. Certainly, diabetes is also no exception from this reason.

Usually, we know that diabetes is from the sugar amount being too much and too high in our body.

Sugar. There are many kinds of sugar in our diet such as fructose, carbohydrate, starch, bread, cake, glucose, and so on. Even if there are so many kinds of sugar, it can be classified into two categories, (1) single sugars and (2) multiple sugars.

A single sugar is one sugar by itself only, such as glucose. A multiple sugar is composed from many different kinds of sugar combined and constructed as another new sugar. This new sugar is a new compound and new chemical, such as carbohydrate, wheat, bread, starch, and others.

Even though are so many sugars around us, diabetes results from only one specific sugar. That is glucose. Thus, an increased amount of sugar in blood can result in diabetes. We have to understand this sugar is glucose.

Diabetes is the high level (amount) of the sugar glucose in our body. Thus, even though there are so many sugars around us and those sugars' amounts are high in our body, surely, those sugars do not have the chance to cause us diabetes at all. By definition, diabetes is a disease for glucose only.

Therefore, multiple sugars can be eaten even in high amounts. Those sugars' levels can still be high in our body, but diabetes cannot be the result of this. This is true.

Even if those sugars' levels are high, it cannot result in the diabetes, but those multiple sugars, after digesting and hydrolyzing, can be changed and converted to the single-sugar form glucose in our body. Then this situation also results in the total amount of glucose being higher. Therefore, eating multiple sugars also plays some role in the occurrence of diabetes.

Now we know the relationship between glucose and diabetes in our body.

How can the glucose amount (level) be high in our body? We must understand the following before we can discuss this.

During ancient times, this disease already existed. Certainly, the treatment by the ancient doctors and medicine was not good at that time. Its treatment at that time certainly was there, but for sure, it was not good. It probably only did some help for those patients.

Since then, treatment methods certainly kept changing and being modified. Knowledge is also continuously improving and updating. Thus, we understand this disease more clearly at this moment. Even if that is true, it is still not that clear now.

I believe that no drug or medicine could be made or synthesized during those periods. The drugs used at the time were all from eating or drinking. They were all from sources that were herbs, plants, insects, or animals. Some of the drugs from those sources would really do little or some help, but some did none at all. Certainly, some sources must have been found there and used as drugs and able to help those suffering from the diseases. Even if there were, those only did a little help against diabetes.

I also believe that it was not until the recent years, wherein the concept of Western medicine was introduced, that patients could be helped. A big changing in the medical field was the result since then. Thus, Western civilization contributed a lot of the success for the treatment of disease.

In those periods, Chinese and Western doctors already knew that a pig's pancreas was able to do some help for this disease when people ate them. However, that was all they knew at that time. Later they might try to eat the contents of the pancreas and also found that the effect was better than eating the whole pancreas alone for diabetes.

They probably also knew that the substance inside the pancreas was the real one that helped heal diabetes. Then after many years later, this inside material of the pancreas probably had been called insulin.

Not until the Westerners introduced the syringe device did the needle get used for injection treatment. After that,

Westerners may have wondered, why not try to put that useful inside material of pancreas, insulin, into the syringe? Then, injecting them to the diabetes patients directly, what could happen? Then they found from the results of this injection that the effect had a big difference and was much better than eating this insulin (inside material of pancreas) alone. After insulin injection, the glucose level in the bloodstream of diabetics can thus be controlled and dropped to normal. However, this situation where the glucose level dropped to normal was not the same case as eating the same amount of insulin. Thus, insulin must be by injection only to be effective, and not by eating. Insulin taken orally is inactive.

Now we understand the relationship between glucose and insulin. Insulin can control the glucose level in our bloodstream.

Why can insulin control the glucose level in the bloodstream?

Before we answer this question, some diabetes patients found after insulin injection treatment that the glucose level in the bloodstream can be controlled to become normal. Without insulin treatment, the glucose level can't be controlled. These situations probably mean that we don't have enough amounts of insulin in our body. So we need the additional amount of insulin introduced into our body to do the job of controlling the glucose level in our body.

Now, the above question is answered. The glucose amount (level) is high in the human body because the insulin level is not enough.

Insulin in the human body is produced by machines (enzymes).

There are many different machines to make many different products and things in the human body. Each of these machines makes its own specific product and thing for maintaining their own specific physiological function and behavior for human life.

However, the ability of each machine to produce the amount of a thing has a limit. Thus, because of this limitation, the amount produced may not be enough or be too much for our body to handle. It is such in insulin production. The glucose level certainly can't be controlled under this condition. Therefore, additional amounts of insulin must be supplied from an external source such as from eating pancreases or from insulin injections.

Unfortunately, later many diabetes patients find that even after insulin injection treatments, it still is useless and no help at all.

From this symptom, we wonder why insulin is not working at all in these diabetes patients. The glucose level still stayed high in bloodstream. From this observation, diabetes can thus be classified into two different kinds:

1. Type 1, insulin-effective diabetes
2. Type 2, insulin treatment inactive

The question here is why insulin treatment is effective in type 1 and not in type 2.

Now we can go back to the question that has been brought up above.

Why can insulin control the glucose level in the bloodstream? If the glucose level can be controlled by insulin, this diabetes patient is a type 1 diabetic.

What is insulin? It is an agent to control the glucose level in the bloodstream.

We can use another way to look at insulin because it is made and produced by the machine in our body. Things or products, after being made by the machines, may look or be treated as an operator. An operator is a worker in the human body. Thus, it can achieve to maintain human physiological functions in a human's life. But the operator must go to its workplace or office to be able to perform its own work. If it can't get into its office, surely, the work can't be done.

Insulin requires doing its work in its office or workplace. It must first travel in the human body, then arrive at its office, and then to do its job.

The office is called the receptor. For easy understanding, the name *receptor* is replaced by *glucose storage* here in this book. The glucose storage is its (insulin's) office.

The glucose storage is clearly a space for storing glucose. Insulin is an operator that does the work of storing the glucose into this storage. The job of insulin is to open the storage door and, thus, enable glucose to flow into the storage. The glucose flowing into the storage space is from the bloodstream. From this pattern and fashion, the amount of glucose in the blood is dropped. The amount of glucose may be continuously reduced, even reaching the normal level. Diabetes symptoms can disappear—no more diabetes there.

Now, it is very clear to us why insulin can let the glucose level drop in human body.

The insufficient amount of insulin in the human body is type 1 diabetes. A syringe injection of external insulin into our body must be required for type 1 diabetes. After the insulin is injected, the external addition of insulin will fix the insulin deficiency situation in the human body to sufficient. Glucose levels thus can be controlled back to the normal in the bloodstream. The diabetes symptoms disappear. This disease is type 1 diabetes.

But we must understand and ask, suppose the case is of both insulin and glucose storage in human body being sufficient enough, is there any possibility the storage door still cannot be opened? If it is, then why can't the door be opened even when both are there and the amounts are also sufficient enough?

This question must be answered as follows:

Suppose there is a door in the room in front of us. If we want to open this door, we must be in the position close by the door. Thus, we are able to open this door. Otherwise, if the distance between the door and us is too far, we will be unable to reach, touch, close, and open this door.

For same reason, if the insulin is far away from the place of the glucose storage, the insulin operator certainly can't reach the storage. Of course, the door can't be opened. Therefore, insulin (operator) must be in the position near the storage door. Then insulin can open the storage door.

After the door is opened by the insulin, the storage door opens; the glucose is able to enter the empty storage space. The glucose level in the bloodstream is thus dropped. The diabetes symptom thus must be not there.

Suppose, in this situation, the door can open and allow glucose to enter this empty storage space. Then why does it not allow the glucose to enter the empty storage to drop glucose levels here? This is a question that can't be explained by medical society.

The only explanation from them is that this diabetes is not the same kind of diabetes. Insulin is useless, and it may have resistance. So this is type 2 diabetes.

Even medical experts can't explain it, but we can bring this question up. Why is it not the same diabetes and having insulin resistance? And why is insulin inactive?

The pharmaceutical company has already made a new drug for this type 2 diabetes. Such a drug has been already on the market and can also be purchased with a prescription.

Even if there is already a drug around for type 2 diabetes treatment, understanding type 2 diabetes is still not quite clear.

I am trying to use a different approach to explain this so-called type 2 diabetes.

Now, assume that we have a pen in our hand and also a paper on the desk. We can use the pen to write the words on this paper. The pen thus acts like an operator, and the pen can do its work writing the words on the paper. The paper thus is an office. If we want to write the words on the paper, the pen must touch the paper. Then we can write the words. Without touching the paper, the words can't be written on the paper by the pen even if both the pen operator and paper office are present there. The work thus can't be done; no words can be written on the paper.

In this circumstance, the pen is the operator and the paper is the office. For the diabetes case, the insulin is an operator and the glucose storage is office. Both the operator and office are coincidentally presented in both of the cases, but they are with different names and not doing the same work in each case. One is writing words, and the other is opening the storage door.

Even if both cases are different from each other, they are both doing the work without any difference. Because circumstances are different, certainly, the works are different. However, the same reasonable reason, if it works for that circumstance, certainly should also be valid and apply to the other circumstance for that work.

If the pen and paper are both there and touching together, the pen can certainly write the words on the paper. However, in this case, if we are not careful enough and drop an oil bottle on this paper, the paper is covered with oil. After the paper is covered with oil, even the oil can be cleaned and wiped out and away from the paper, there will still be oil marks remaining on the paper. Under this situation, in no way can words be written on this paper anymore. The words can't be written on this oil-covered paper. Thus, work certainly can't be performed and accomplished here.

The pen and paper are both still there; both can also be touched, but words cannot be written on the paper. It just means that in this situation of the "operator" pen and "office" paper, even if both are there, the work can't be done. It is just as the case in the inactive insulin situation, where both insulin and the storage are there. But the door can't be opened. And the work can't be done. These situations are no different.

Why can't words be written?

Words can't be written anymore, because even if the pen touches the paper's surface, it doesn't truly touch the paper at all. There is an oil layer covering the surface of the paper. The oil layer is present between the paper and the pen. It thus results in the paper having no chance to touch the tip of the pen. The tip of the pen only touches the oil layer on the paper. Words certainly can't be written on the paper. The pen thus cannot do the work of writing.

However, the pen is still working. It still can write words on paper, but only in the case, oil is not there. Therefore, the pen (operator) is OK, and nothing is wrong. Words can't be written because the paper (office) is covered by the oil layer. This is the reason the words can't be written. And it is not from the reason of the paper and pen both being bad. Therefore, the words can't be written on the paper because of the oil layer in between the paper and pen.

Thus, this explanation makes perfect sense to know why words can't be written (work can't be performed).

Can we apply this reason and explanation to the "operator and office" (insulin and sugar storage) circumstance there?

This same reason applies to the situation of operator (insulin) and office (glucose storage), It may be explained as follows:

In the diabetes case of the "operator and office" (insulin and glucose storage) circumstance, insulin can open the door of glucose storage. After the door is opened, the glucose can enter into this storage. Certainly, the glucose level in the blood must drop and be reduced. If the amount of glucose in the blood decreases and reaches the normal level, the diabetes symptom is reduced or disappears from our body.

However, in the case of the "operator and office" (insulin and glucose storage), in the problem, malfunction, or something similar, there is supposedly another thing, material, or chemical present between them. Thus, this thing will block the contact between the insulin and the storage. Contact blocked, the storage door certainly can't be opened. The storage room will be completely empty. The door cannot open; the glucose surely can't enter the glucose storage room. The glucose level definitely can't be dropped and reduced. The diabetes symptoms still remain. This is the same reason, same mechanism, and identical phenomenon as the pen and paper circumstance when words can't be written on paper. They are the same and no different.

Whether this reason and explanation are true or not, certainly, applying this concept to the diabetes patients is still a big question.

Even if it is correct, it still needs to be proven. This kind of proof is usually obtained from clinical studies by the pharmaceutical industry or hospital. However, there is no chance to have this clinical study to be done by them.

For doing a clinical study, it requires tremendous manpower, huge revenue, and time. At the end, it may end up with nothing and may not be worth doing.

Besides, even if clinical studies are done just to test a reason or an idea, even if it is found correct, there is no standby product. Thus, the theory or idea cannot be on the market to sell as a drug or product. No benefit can be earned, and no profit can be made from this at all. It, thus, is worthless for the pharmaceutical industry to do the clinical study. A new drug is invented as a product that can be sold and make huge profits. Therefore, a clinical study is for the drug (product) only and not for the theory or concept at all. The pharmaceutical industry certainly will not do it, this clinical study.

Question: what thing is between "insulin and glucose storage"?

This will be mentioned a little later.

In the recent forty-year period, maybe shorter or longer, hospitals and doctors' offices found that many diabetes patients automatically recovered by nature. Glucose levels dropped to normal, and diabetes symptoms disappeared. They observed no clue and explanation for why diabetes symptoms were gone from them. Many years later, they even found more: those recovered diabetics were all type 2 patients. That was all they knew, but why, they still can't answer.

Many years later, they also found that those recovered type 2 patients all were classified as overweight, obese, and fat persons. Overweight means the body is loaded with a lot of fat, oil, and cholesterol in the body. Later they also found that after those type 2 patients lost their weight, diabetes symptoms were gone naturally. Thus, those observations collected from hospitals and medical offices make us understand that those naturally recovered diabetes patients are all type 2 patients and they also are overweight.

After losing weight, diabetes symptoms disappeared. It is certainly clear to let us know that when an obese person becomes skinny, diabetes symptoms disappears. It also means that the glucose level is dropped to normal. Losing weight here means oily substances are moved to the outside of our body. The oily substances are removed and gone. We recover from diabetes. This is a very strong evidence indicating that the things that are in between the insulin and the glucose storage are the oily substances.

Even this is not from clinical study. But it is strong enough to prove my point that the other thing is the oily substance in between the insulin and storage. The oily substances (fat and cholesterol) block the contact between the glucose storage and the insulin. Thus insulin can't touch the storage to open the door. Thus it can't let the glucose enter the storage space. Then the glucose level stays high in the bloodstream. Diabetes is surely occurring.

Thus, this claimed type 2 diabetes is not the same as normal diabetes because insulin is useless for this diabetes and also probably considering there is resistance occurring to the insulin. After being explained here, those claims are not correct. Type 2 diabetes is still directly related to the situation of the insulin "operator" and glucose storage "office" here.

We should keep in our mind that both the insulin and the glucose storage are still OK and nothing is wrong with them in human body.

Thus, type 2 diabetes is very clear to us. It is from too much oily substances presently in our body.

Now it is clear that

1. type 2 diabetes results from too much oily substances in the body;
2. type 1 diabetes results from a lack of insulin in the body.

Even if the occurrence of type 1 is caused by an insufficient amount of *insulin*, is there any chance that type 1 diabetes is also possible from the reason of *oily substances*?

Yes, it is possible. The amount of oily substances may also contribute to type 1 diabetes. Even if this consideration has not been proven yet, it's possible that it is still there. However, we can still bring this question here. If this question and answer are reasonable, even if it is not proven, the possibility still could be there. It may require proving in near future.

The amount of oily substances (oil, fat, and cholesterol) in the body may result to two different environments: (1) too much or overloaded, or (2) a low amount present.

Overloading oily substances results in type 2 diabetes. We already know that.

Even if there are fewer amounts of oily substances in the body, it still can bind to and block some of the glucose storage to make a storage shortage. Thus some storage spaces are missing and gone. This storage shortage is just as the situation of the insulin operator amount not being enough. Thus, type 1 symptoms are also possible from low amounts of oily substances (oil, fat, and cholesterol) blocking the storage.

In this case, this diabetes (possible type 1) is from storage shortage, and it is not from the insulin amount not being enough.

The reason even it is for the situation of storage shortage, storage shortage meant available number of storage door can be opened by insulin less. But the total amount of storage in the body are remaining the same no change.

The number of storage reduced even though the insulin amount is enough there. But the total binding force from that amount of insulin is not necessarily strong enough to compete with those fewer amounts of oily substances bound to the storage. Thus, not all storage doors can be opened. The glucose level surely can't be dropped enough. The disease diabetes is, therefore, also here. Therefore, additional amount of insulin is also required here. In this situation, the available storage shortage, thus, is also possibly resulting as the amount of insulin is not enough there. They are no different. Both situations, thus, are type 1 diabetes.

The situation of the available storage amount shortage is also as type 1 diabetes. Its reason can be explained as the following:

Oily substances cover the storage surface because they are binding there. Thus, they can bind together. Binding requires binding affinity between them. The binding and binding affinity also are occurring between the insulin and glucose storage too. The binding affinity for the oily substances or for the insulin binding to the storage is not the same, not identical. Surely, it is different. For sure, one must be greater than the other. In case of the binding affinity, the oily substances are better than the insulin in binding to the storage. The insulin has a lesser chance to bind to the storage compared with oily substances. Thus, this situation of storage shortage certainly is here. Surely, insulin here is partially inactive.

To make insulin fully active again, we can try and use the method below:

As an example, if an adult is standing by the door and blocking it, a child can't pass this door. The child certainly is not strong and powerful enough to push this adult away from this door. The force of one child may be not strong enough to push this adult away from this door.

Nevertheless, if many children group together, the combined force must be strong enough. Certainly, the adult can be pushed away from this door. And the door is opened, and the children can pass through.

This reason can be applied to the situation of insulin and oily substances binding to the storage cases. Even the binding affinity between the insulin and storage is much weaker than between the oily substances and storage.

Naturally, even if the amount of the internal insulin is enough in the body, the binding affinity from this amount might not be strong enough against the low amount of oily substances binding to the storage. Thus, the oily substances are still able to bind to the storage. However, the syringe injects an additional amount of insulin to the body. The total amount from the natural internal insulin and plus the external insulin the syringe injected together—these two amounts together are certainly enough and able to increase the power and force for the binding. Then the oily substances can be pushed out and away from the surface of the glucose storage. Thus, the insulin can reach and bind to the storage. Therefore, the door can be opened. Now the insulin becomes active, and it is effective. This symptom here is just as in the type 1 symptom from insufficient insulin situation (requires additional external insulin supplied). Thus this diabetes occurring is from fewer amounts of oily substances here that are bound to the certain amount of storage, then it is resulting to the shortage. Thus, it is also possible and can be considered as type 1. It is also as the situation requiring additional external insulin supplied.

For type 2, overloading oily substances, even if a syringe injects external amounts of insulin into the body, those additional amounts from external injection are still not necessarily more than enough. It is compared with the overloaded amount of oily substances there. Thus, it is still unable to increase the binding affinity and force for insulin. The oily substances, thus, can't be pushed away from the storage surface. It thus still is useless. It still is type 2 diabetes.

In the other kind of diabetes, the amount of insulin produced is not enough in the body; certainly, it is the factor resulting in type 1 diabetes. In addition, the decreased amount of oily substances covering the storage door can also contribute to type 1 diabetes in patients. Even though this situation is not confirmed yet in the medical society, the possibility is still there. For the time being, we can't rule this possibility out for type 1 diabetes.

If we don't want to have diabetes, we should change our eating habits to control the amount of sugar (glucose) and oily substances together to a suitable level in our body. We should keep this in our mind. Thus, the diabetes can be avoided in our life.

Type 1 diabetes is also possible from a low amount of oily substances present in humans.

Chapter 7

Three High

"Three high" is a disease. Usually, symptoms occur only as one disease in patients. However, for the three high disease, it is different. It is three different kinds of diseases all found together in the same patient. These three different diseases found are high blood pressure, high cholesterol, and high sugar.

As discussed in chapters 1 and 2, these diseases can occur in us from our eating habits, by eating too much. Too much food eaten enters our body. The food collected and cumulated in our body surely results to the amount or level changed from normal (suitable) to high or too high. If the amount is higher than normal in the body, the disease certainly occurs as a result. Too much of each food in the body results in its own responsive disease occurring. For the three high disease, its occurrence is from three different diets with exceeding amounts. They are salt, sugar, and cholesterol—all three amounts high.

Therefore, this three high disease is also no exception. It is also caused by eating too much. But this three high disease happens only from too much of one special food. *Only this one food can cause these three different diseases occurring together in the same patient.*

This food is cholesterol (oily substances). If we eat too much, the amount of cholesterol in our body results to the level going from normal to high or much higher. Thus, in our body, the first disease occurs. It is high cholesterol (first high) disease.

Cholesterol, if too much in our body, sticks on the blood vessels and builds up the plaque there. After plaque is built up, the opening for the blood flowing in the vessel is smaller. The space for flowing blood is smaller. The flowing blood is slowed down in the vessel.

Blood moves and flows slowly, thus triggering the occurrence of higher blood pressure. High blood pressure thus happens—the second disease occurs in our body. This is the second high (high blood pressure) disease. Even if this is the second disease, the second high, it is from the same thing: caused by too much of the same food (cholesterol) in the human body.

However, cholesterol is not necessarily only sticking to the blood vessel. It also sticks to other places. For example, the glucose storage place—if this occurs, the storage surface is packed and covered by the large amount of cholesterol there. Therefore, the glucose storage is unable to be reached and touched by the operator insulin. The operator (insulin) certainly can't open the storage door anymore. The glucose amount, therefore, is high in the bloodstream. The glucose level should stay high. Thus, the third disease happens to the same human body. This is the third high in our body. It is high sugar disease.

Thus, even though three different "high diseases" are found in the same patient, it still is from the same source, caused by too much of the same material found in the food. It is cholesterol.

Patients quite worry about the disease of three high. However, patients just need to control their eating habits to minimize the amount of oily substances from the food intake daily. Soon the amount of cholesterol reaches back to normal. The symptoms of the three high disease can either be minimized, be improved, or disappear. If we don't try to change our eating habits to help us eliminate the disease, then no one can help us. Remember, only you yourself can help you do it.

Chapter 8

Irregular Heartbeat

The EKG (electrocardiogram) technique can diagnose your heart condition—whether it is in the normal heartbeat pattern or not. If it does not have a normal pattern, the atrial fibrillation symptom may be found in your body. Doctors will usually treat you with a blood thinner medicine. It will lessen the thickness of your blood's consistency in your body. Thus, your blood can flow easily in the blood vessel.

Another reason is that if blood becomes thicker, then the condition of the blood will be more concentrated and heavier. The more concentrated it is, the more the blood's original function will also alter differently from its normal situation, especially since, after being concentrated, the blood's volume is lessened. Blood volume here is very important. The job of the blood's amount is bringing the oxygen in and then carrying it over to the heart. The increased amount of blood can cause more oxygen to be brought in to the heart too.

The condition of higher concentration will also influence the situation of blood circulation. Oxygen is the energy. If it brings in less amounts of oxygen, the force, energy, and power applied to the heart certainly cannot be adequate. The heartbeat and circulation, thus, will not function well in the heart.

If the blood becomes thinner, the blood volume will be in the normal condition; the deficiency situation of oxygen, energy, force, and power certainly is not occurring. Thus, heartbeat and circulation will function normally in the heart.

When atrial fibrillation occurs, it usually is generating *the heartbeat in an irregular pattern* (irregular heart rhythm).

The irregular heartbeat pattern is possibly caused by the situation of thicker blood occurring. The blood, if thicker, is certainly more concentrated; the blood volume is also less than before. It is just as the situation where the amount of blood in the heart is not enough. When the amount of blood is not enough in the heart, the oxygen is also not enough in the heart. Thus, the heart can't have enough force and energy there. The heartbeat isn't normal. *The irregular pattern* can happen.

We may use a different approach to explain its occurrence.

The heart requires beating. Beating requires the force, energy, and power in the heart and in our body to do this function. People usually find that the force, energy, and power are not enough when they are getting old. But they are not necessarily aware of this situation occurring in them. This lack of force can, on rare occasions, also happen to younger and middle-aged people. Those situations in the human body can also result in an abnormal heartbeat pattern.

The force, energy, and power in the human body come from water and food. Therefore, if water and food amounts are not enough in the human body, the force, energy, and power are also insufficient for the heart to beat normally.

The insufficient amount of food and water in the human body is usually found in older-aged persons. But they are not necessarily aware of this situation. Thus the normal possible heartbeat pattern cannot be achieved by them, and it possibly results in their irregular heartbeat.

Why is the insufficient situation of force, energy, and power in the heart?

As mentioned above, the reason generally found is old age. At old age, those conditions of water amount insufficiency and hunger usually happen to them.

Hunger relates to the situation of an empty stomach. Dehydration relates to the case of a lesser blood amount in the heart.

When a human body feels weak, it means that it doesn't have enough force and energy to use. Thus the body tells you to fix this problem. It thus requires you to get energy from an external source, from outside your body. It thus lets you know that the body is hungry. Then humans require eating food to supply the energy to their body. Hunger is a natural phenomenon to inform you that the force and energy in your body are not enough. So weakness is a sign of the condition of hunger.

In other words, with the lack of blood amount in the system, the blood circulation certainly is not performing well too. Air, oxygen, is energy. It can be brought into the heart by blood from the lungs. The amount of air and oxygen that can be brought in strictly depends on the amount of blood there. An increased amount of blood can bring in more air and oxygen into the heart. The more oxygen is brought in, the more energy can be generated in the heart. Vice versa, with less blood, certainly less air and oxygen can be brought in. Then less energy can be generated in the heart. The more amounts of oxygen brought in, the more the force to trigger the heartbeat is increased. The irregular heartbeat situation possibly is not occurring.

In old people, usually their blood amounts are not sufficient. They don't know it. The insufficient blood situation is usually from the case of lacking water in their body.

Why is water lacking?

Old people can't hold that much amounts of water in the body. Even if they drink a large amount of and enough water daily, they can't hold their water long enough. Usually, the situation of an insufficient amount of water is occurring in them. Therefore, the force, energy, and power are also certainly inadequate in their body.

In the blood, the larger portion of its components is water. The more water in the body, the more blood will be there too. More air and oxygen can be brought in too. More force, energy, and power surely can be generated there in the heart also. Thus, the heart will have enough force to beat. If the force, energy, and power are insufficient there in the heart, the irregular heartbeat is also possible in the heart. Thus, water is a very important factor in maintaining higher or lower blood amount in the heart.

As mentioned above, even if the situation of hunger and insufficient water occurs in their body, they are not necessarily able to know that this situation is already occurring to them. Sometimes even when they know that this situation (requiring them to eat food and drink water) is already occurring to them, they don't worry and don't care at all or just ignore it.

For irregular heartbeat situation

Sometimes the rate of heartbeat is much faster than normal. Sometimes it is much less than normal. Sometimes, the tension for the heart to beat is so weak, and sometimes the heartbeat stops midbeat. Those symptoms will generally be found when there is an irregular heartbeat.

If the heartbeat found is missing in the middle, it is because the heart doesn't have enough force and energy.

The heartbeat requires a certain amount of force and energy. If there is no force and no energy, the heart certainly can't beat and pump. If there is no heartbeat there, the human, no question, will die. Thus a certain fixed amount of force and energy must be there for the heart to beat all the time in your life.

Because of this reason, the total fixed amount of force and energy must be present there. Those forces must apply to each heartbeat, for about 60 beats in each minute, respectively. The heart must provide these forces. In most cases, the fixed total amount of the forces is supposedly only enough to provide the 60 beats in a minute. Usually, this is for the normal pattern for heart function. Now change the heartbeat's rate: it is from the normal 60 beats per minute to 120 beats per minute. This fixed total amount of force originally is supplied for 60 beats in a minute. Now it is changed; it is provided and distributed to the new pattern of 120 beats per minute. This force there, thus, is certainly not adequate as usual for each beat. Thus the heart, the heartbeat, is very weak. This weak situation is also found in the wrist's pulse feeling.

The fixed amount of force for 60 beats per minute now changes to the 120 beats per minute. Two issues must require consideration for performing the heartbeat function. It is the timing for the heart to beat time. The other also is the timing, but instead it is for the energy (force) built up in the heart and then applied to the beat for pumping. These two different timings must match with each other to perform the normal heartbeat pattern. If these two different timings cannot match with each other, if either timing is missing or it is not arriving on time for the other timing, the beat function certainly can't be performed well and occur in the heart. Suppose the timing for heart beating time is arriving already but the energy (force) built up is not there for the other timing. The heartbeat certainly can't occur. Vice versa, if the timing for energy (force) built up is arriving but the heart beating time is not there, it is also true. The heartbeat certainly can't perform well.

If this situation is in the middle of heartbeat, the heartbeat will certainly not occur.

From the above considerations, in the heartbeat with this new 120-beats-per-minute pattern, the heart is only receiving half the full force from the original 60-beats-per-minute pattern. Thus, this half-full force may apply to several individual beats in this new pattern (fast heartbeat rate pattern). But some of the beats may even not receive any force and energy at all. If this situation is in the middle of the heartbeat, the pulse disappearing midbeat would certainly occur. Thus the faster rate of the heartbeat would result to the disappearing midbeat. The missed pulse and irregular heartbeat situations are also generally found in fast-heartbeat rate patients. This condition is usually found in older people.

Thus, this insufficient situation is possibly from an inadequate water amount and an empty stomach. People, especially the elderly, must be aware of this. Therefore, we must drink a lot of water and eat more food frequently to minimize the occurrence of this abnormal heart situation.

Chapter 9

Pain

Pain is a typical feeling symptom. It's usually at a local area in our body. The nervous system is also involved in feeling pain.

Pain is usually felt after being injured. It is usually found in local areas such as the places where your body has been hit, beat, or others. In those areas, the environment and the configuration are changed. The symptoms of expanding and constricting also happen there as a result. Thus, an unfavorable and different feeling will result in those areas. This special one, this uncomfortable feeling, is called pain. Pain is also a sickness.

Pain involves the nervous system. For example, if we sharply cut the hand away at the wrist from the arm, then the hand and the arm will not connect there together as one piece. The hand and wrist are not connected anymore. Thus, the pain is only at the position of the wrist's wound. But pain is not in the hand at all even though the areas of the wound are at both the hand and wrist.

Why? After cutting the wrist, it is still connected with the arm and our body. So the nerves also connect to the wrist wound. Because nerves are connected, we have a painful feeling in the wrist. But after being cut off, the hand does not connect anymore with body; the nerves certainly don't connect with the hand anymore. The painful feeling from the hand certainly can't happen there.

If the hand doesn't completely cut away from the wrist, the hand still partially connects with the wrist and also with our body. In this case, the wound in the hand part thus also feels terribly painful. Thus, pain is not just in the hand area. Certainly, it also includes the wrist area. In this situation, the hand certainly feels pain. It is because of the nerves in the hand still connecting to the body; thus, both hand and wrist feel pain together.

Therefore, feeling pain must relate to the nerves, but nerves must connect together to make it happen. Without nerves there and connecting, pain surely would not happen.

With the hand, wrist, and body connecting together, the nerves also connect together there. Thus, the message of pain can be sent out, back and forth from each other.

The feeling of pain involves two different functions of the nervous system. These two functions there result in pain. Question—why is pain only in the wounded area and not in some other places after an injury?

From these two functions, the first one, at the wound area, the nerves at the wrist area send their wound information to the central nervous zone. They tell the central zone where this message is sent from and what happened here. The central nervous area in the brain receives this message. Then the central nervous system sends back a message to the wound of the wrist area. It then lets the wrist area to know that the wound is occurring there. After the wounded area receives this returning message, because only the wounded area received this returning message, pain occurs, and certainly, it only occurs in the wrist area of the wound. The pain, thus, is not occurring in other places. The returned message also includes how to treat this wound information, such as more heat being there and also more fluid flowing into this wound. This function is a natural way to treat and fix this wound on our body for the pain. Thus, this wounded wrist area is very hot and swollen.

If the hand is cut away, there are no nerves connecting it to the arm at all. If no nerves are connected, certainly, the injury message cannot be transferred, sent, and returned from each other, between these two areas. Thus there is no painful feeling in the wounded area of the cut-off hand.

How can we know that these message transmissions function? They are involved in the local nerves to the central nervous system back and forth. And how can we be so sure that it is not from the other reason?

The first message must be sent out from the wound, then to the central nervous system. If this message is blocked, no information can be delivered. The second returning message surely can't be returned and delivered to the wound area. If no message is received, certainly, no pain can be felt.

Because no pain can be felt, this transferring function certainly is not occurring in our body; it is already proven in the situation where the hand is cut off. It also indicates that the nerves are not connected there.

No nerves connect between the hand (cut away) and our body. Messages certainly can't transfer from each other. Thus, no pain will be in the hand. If both of them still connect together, messages definitely can be received. The hand certainly will feel pain.

Using another example to explain, we can use painkilling drugs to minimize the painful feeling in the wound area or inject it with anesthetic medicine to make the pain go. After using these kinds of medicine, the painful feeling is either minimized or gone. The pain may not be there anymore, but the nerves are still connecting.

In this situation, the nerves are still connecting between each other. The pain is gone because the message and information can't be transferred anymore because of this medicine treatment. The nerve function is blocked by the medicine treatment; the nerve-transferring function is not occurring. No messages can be delivered and transferred; thus, no place can receive the message. The painful feeling is certainly not there and not occurring.

In the chapter on strokes, we already mentioned that the *message can be considered as merchandise*. Merchandise transfer requires energy to make this delivery situation in our body. The *nerve* is the human cable that also acts as a traffic *highway*. It is for energy transporting messages in human body. *Energy is oxygen* from the blood and also functions *as a vehicle*. If there is no energy supplied or no vehicle there, the message certainly cannot be transferred and delivered in the human body. The pain certainly can't happen in the human body.

However, even if energy (vehicle) is there, if it is blocked by the medicine treatment, the transporting function certainly can't be performed. Information can't be delivered to each other. Pain, thus, will not happen and be gone.

Thus it is clear to us that the occurrence of pain directly involves the nervous system.

Pain. In case you expect the feeling of pain to be reduced in your body, the best thing to do is change your current environment. Surround yourself with a different one and not the present one. When the environment changes, message also changes, and the painful feeling also changes.

Changing the environment, in this case, must depend on the exercise performed. However, if you only do walking exercise, it certainly can't help you reduce your pain too much. There is also the fact that most persons will reject doing exercise because of pain. If you can continue to do the exercise despite the pain there, at the end, the results after exercise will definitely be different, and the feeling of pain is certainly reduced tremendously too. If you can do this exercise daily, after a long time the pain will certainly not happen easily to you.

With a change in environment, the pain information and message (for delivering and transporting) are also changed. The original pain message is now changed to a different one after exercise. Because it is different and not the original pain message, the original pain message certainly can't be received. Instead, the nerves receive a different message. If the message is different, certainly, the painful feeling is different, and possibly, no pain will be felt there. Pain is definitely reduced or gone.

Chapter 10

Lastly, Be Aware; It May Save Your Life

We will all die sooner or later in the near future. However how and when we die are different from one to another. Some die from sickness, some from accidents, some from murder, some from suicide, some from drowning, and some from natural events such as earthquakes, hurricanes, and others.

Death from sickness can result from hypertension, heart attack, stroke, diabetes, and others. The symptom of every disease is different. Therefore, the situation of death is different from each other.

The conditions of dying are different from one another. But the question is, are the conditions of death the same or not?

The answer from us is probably yes, but the condition is different. Final death is when a body no longer breathes.

Most of you probably consider this the case resulting in death. If there is no breath, certainly, death will occur. This is true.

In fact, final death is not from not breathing. This answer is incorrect.

It is when the heart stops pumping (beating). If the heart is no longer beating, blood then stops circulating. No oxygen and energy can be supplied from the blood to our body anymore. If there is no energy, no heartbeat could be there, and certainly, we would die.

If there is no heartbeat, there is no breath too. Thus not breathing is from the heart not beating.

Why is it not from the stopped breath but from the stopped heartbeat?

For example, when a dying person is brought back to life again, usually, he is saved by a member of the emergency medical team. The procedure to save his life is by CPR (cardiopulmonary resuscitation) techniques. Doing CPR requires you to blow the air into the body, the lungs first, of the nearly dead person. After the air is blown into his lungs, he is still remaining in death and is not yet alive. Even though the air is already in the lungs, breath still cannot happen and life is not occurring too.

Not until his heart is pushed, then his heart starts to beat again. Then he survives and is alive again. The lungs also begin to breathe again. It is thus clear to us and also tells us that if there is no heartbeat there, certainly, there is also no breath. It is still dead. Therefore, the final symptom of death is when the heart is not beating, and it is not when the lungs are not breathing.

We always hear that someone just died while he was doing his work in his backyard. We also hear some die while climbing on a mountain, some while walking on the street, some on the exercise machine, some on the bicycle, and some even while having sex, and others. In all these situations where death happens, the medical society considers it as a heart attack. We also agree with it. It is from heart attack.

On further consideration, I myself do not totally agree with this conclusion. The death is not from a heart attack. It is from the condition where there is no more force and power supply to the heart to trigger it to pump and beat. The heart doesn't have enough force and energy there; certainly, the heart can't do the action of heartbeat well. When the heartbeat stops, death occurs.

Even this situation is from this reason. The person's death is because of not having enough force and energy. However, when they work at that moment, they are not necessarily aware that they are already in this situation. Therefore, they continue to do their work. Thus, the remaining force and energy in their body are consumed and spent on the work. The leftover force and energy becomes less and less. It may even be reduced at the risk of being unable to survive in that condition. Death will finally occur.

For survival, in this situation, the body's defense system will automatically promote the ability to increase the force and energy a little more. After increasing force, it enables us to continue to do the work.

This increasing force is from the heart; it is from an increased heartbeat rate. When the heartbeat rate is increased, the heart's blood pressure is also increased as a response. When the blood pressure is increased, the amount of force and energy in our body thus is also automatically increased.

Because the amount of force and energy is increased, this increased force in our body will allow our work to be continued. The force and energy are even increased here; however, it is also a result of a faster heartbeat rate.

Unfortunately, we still keep continuing to do the work without trying to stop.

The force is kept consumed for this backyard work. After this cycle is repeated many times, it finally can't be further repeated. It makes the force and energy less and less until it is finally completely gone from our body. Thus our body has no more force there. No more force can be increased anymore. The heartbeat is surely stopped, thus resulting in death.

The heart stops pumping and beating. With no heartbeat, death occurs. This is the reason why those people died on their work. Therefore, those people did not necessarily die from heart attacks. It is because their hearts stopped pumping and beating.

Another situation

When you are at home alone, suddenly, *if you don't feel well*, is there any possibility for you to diagnose and find out what happened to you at that moment?

It is difficult, and even if you go to a hospital, it may require many steps to find out and also should take more times to know what caused it.

However, if this situation is really happening to you at home, you should do the following steps, and also call your doctor if you can.

You should lie and sit down first, then (1) check your blood pressure and (2) check your pulse at your wrist.

1. Checking your blood pressure

It requires you to have a blood pressure gauge to monitor it. Usually, it can be done at home. If you are not at home and are outside, certainly, you can't bring the blood pressure monitor with you there. Therefore, you can't measure your blood pressure at that moment. The blood pressure-measuring step certainly can't be performed outside. Measuring the blood pressure is only applied in case you are home.

After measuring your blood pressure, if it is high, usually, you will find yourself feeling dizzy. The dizzy feeling is also found in low-blood pressure patients. However, the dizziness found is quite different between people with high and low blood pressures.

The dizzy situation occurs in a high-blood pressure patient, but the body is very strong. In the low-blood pressure patient, besides the dizzy feeling, the symptom of weakness also happens in this person's body. Especially in this situation, your head feels terribly faint immediately after bowing then returning to the standing position. But in this situation, this dizzy feeling is never found in normal or high-blood pressure persons.

2. Check the pulse at your wrist

This check is more important than measuring blood pressure.

Certainly, after checking the pulse, you will know your heart condition at present—whether it is strong or weak and the heartbeat normal or not. However, we have no way to touch the heart to determine it. Instead we can check the pulse at the wrist to replace checking on the heart directly.

Because there is a heartbeat in the heart, there is also a pulse beating at the wrist. They are identical, not different. Thus, checking the pulse at the wrist surely is also the same as checking your heart's present conditions. This is a valid method to find out whether your heart is in the normal condition or not. Thus the pulse's beat is the heartbeat; there is no difference from each other. But checking on the pulse must be done with our finger and not by a device.

After checking on your wrist, it tells you that your heartbeat is fast or slow. It also lets you know if there is any beat missing in the heart or not. Besides that, it also shows if the heartbeat is strong or weak.

From those observations, we can obtain a lot of our heart's information the moment we are not feeling well.

If the heartbeat (pulse beat) is slow, it usually means the heartbeat is weak. Certainly, wrist pulse beat is also slow. Thus, it lets us know that the heart doesn't have enough force (energy) to beat.

If the heartbeat (pulse beat) is faster, it also tells us that the same situation of insufficient power and force is in the heart. However, with lacking power in the heart, the heartbeat usually slows down initially. But for surviving, the defense system raises the rate of heartbeat faster from slower. Thus, this is the reason why the heartbeat (pulse beat) found is faster in humans in this situation. Therefore, a faster heartbeat means the heart is in a bad condition and has insufficient power and force. Surely, the heart is beating abnormally.

The heart doesn't have enough force and power. Why is it so?

The pulse beat, if weak, is slow, fast, or missed in the middle. You must watch out yourself to avoid the serious risk that may happen to you.

If the heartbeat is missing in the middle, that also means that the situation of insufficient force, energy, and power is in the heart already.

The heartbeat requires a certain amount of force and energy there to trigger the heart to beat. If the force and energy are not enough there, the heart certainly can't function well. An abnormal heartbeat pattern must be there. Seriously, there is no question that a human will die because of this. Thus, a certain fixed amount of force and energy must be there for the heart to beat all the time in your life.

The irregular heartbeat is discussed in chapter 8. The details for the weak, fast, slow, and missed pulse situations are all already explained there.

When there is not enough force (energy or power) in the heart, surely, it is from either situations of insufficient water or hunger in the body. Possibly, both situations can also happen together. Thus, we must try to save our force and energy in our body and also keep this idea in the mind for our own good.

After your blood pressure and pulse have been checked, you should be aware of your heart condition. Then you should lie or sit down to save the force staying in your body.

Next we must fix this situation of not feeling well.

The following two things should be done immediately. It may save your life.

1. Drinking a lot of water and liquid

    What thing is in the heart? It is blood. There is also the function of blood circulation in the human body. Blood can bring a lot of things, circulating together with it, to every part of our body, including the heart. One of those things brought along with the blood is oxygen from the lungs. The oxygen brought in by the blood then circulates together with it all over our body.

    In the blood, the major component is water. If the water amount is not enough in our body, our blood amount also is not enough in the heart. Surely, blood circulation is not well; certainly, it is not good for the heart at all. Besides, if blood amount is not enough, the amount of oxygen that can be carried and brought in, of course, is also not enough. If oxygen and energy are not enough, the force in the heart is also not adequate to trigger the normal heartbeat function. Therefore, the heart can't beat well too.

    To fix this problem, we must drink a lot of water and liquids. After we drink a lot of water and liquids, the water and liquid amounts are increased in our body. It follows that a higher amount of water is also entering the heart. Thus the blood amount is also increased naturally.

If the blood amount is increased in the heart, definitely, the blood circulation and functions are also well and much better than before. Besides that, the higher the blood amount, the more oxygen is also brought to the heart. The more oxygen there is in the heart, the more the force to beat the heart increases, stronger than before. The heartbeat pattern will surely be better and may change back to the normal. This is the reason why we should drink a lot of water or liquids.

2.   Eating more food

When our body feels very weak, it means an insufficient force can be found in the human body. Surely, food must be supplied to fix this hunger problem. Naturally, the stomach will let us know that hunger is happening to us. Thus, we must eat more food.

In some circumstances, for some persons, they feel hungry even after they just ate. This symptom is hard to be explained. It is because that heart doesn't have enough force there to beat. No force or no energy in the heart automatically results in the feeling of intense hunger.

After eating, the force and energy are increased in our body. The heart, thus, also has enough force to beat. The normal heartbeat pattern may also be achieved. This is the reason why we must eat more food.

Thus, when the situation of not feeling well happens at home, to survive, the heart is required to beat. Enough force must be present there in the heart. Therefore, we must drink a lot of water and liquids and also eat more food immediately to fix this situation. It is very important. Therefore, bringing a lot of food and more water outside with you is a necessary step.

Usually, (1) the blood is not adequate, not enough, and (2) the stomach is hungry. These situations often occur in old people, but they are not aware it's occurring in their body. Certainly, it is a very serious and dangerous situation to them.

After both situations of "more food and water" are accomplished in our body, the heartbeat's function can definitely be performed much better. The feeling of being unwell will probably change back to normal. Possibly, the life also can be saved.

Conclusion

Health and disease are very important and serious issues to human life. Even it is true. There are many different diseases around us. Humans know about some of them, but some are still not clear at all to us.

Even though this situation is there, time keeps changing to the future. The understanding of diseases today is better than the past. However, even if knowledge is updated and improving, it is still very limited. To know all of them, theoretically, is impossible.

Humans understand illness well enough these days. Human knowledge of illness from the past is now quite extensive globally. Even though the combined knowledge is quite enough, we are still too far away from understanding. Certainly, humans can't explain everything. Human knowledge is very limited. However, everything in nature has a reason. Nothing is without reason in nature. It can all be explained. Unfortunately, because of our limited knowledge now (combined from the past and global), humans can't explain most things at this moment. It definitely can be explained later in the near future or after a longer period of time.

Health and disease are part of nature. Nature is too broad, too huge. It is impossible for humans to know and solve all natural phenomena. At least humans can do something: keep improving and updating to know them more and more. But it is impossible to know all nature, even in the near future.

References

Cheung, Hong Son. 1998. *Hypertension and Rational Design of Captopril, the First ACE Inhibitor for the Treatment of Hypertension*. Rockville, MD: Kabel Publishers.

Cheung, Hong Son. 2009. *The Mystery of Hypertension*. Bloomington, IN: Xlibris Corporation.

Cheung, Hong Son (張洪聲). 2009. 解琵高血壓之謎 [The mystery of hypertension]. Taipei, Taiwan: 橘井文化事業股份有限公司.

Cushman, D. W. and H. S. Cheung. 1971. "Spectrophotometric assay and properties of the angiotensin-converting enzyme of rabbit lung," *Biochemical Pharmacology* 20: 1637-1648

Index

www.ingramcontent.com/pod-product-compliance
Lightning Source LLC
Chambersburg PA
CBHW030816180526
45163CB00003B/1311